NO GALLBLADDER DIET COOKBOOK

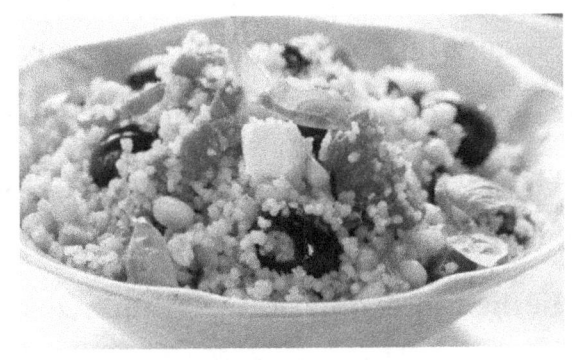

A Comprehensive Guide to Healthy Living with Low-Fat Recipes and Digestive-Friendly Meals After Gallbladder Removal

KELLY C. BROWN

CONTENTS

INTRODUCTION

Clara, a vivacious and health-conscious woman, was confronted with the prospect of living without her gallbladder following a necessary surgical procedure. Determined to live a healthy lifestyle, she researched nutrition and learned the importance of a well-balanced diet adapted to her individual requirements.

Clara embraced the experience, exploring numerous resources and discovering a great companion—the "No Gallbladder Diet Cookbook." This cookbook became her go-to resource, providing a wealth of delicious meals meant to help digestion without placing her digestive system under stress.

Clara felt a revitalized sense of well-being after including nutrient-dense foods and attentive meal planning. Her breakfasts included fiber-rich oats, fresh fruits, and low-fat yogurt, guaranteeing a continuous flow of energy throughout the day. Lunches and dinners included lean foods such as grilled chicken and fish, as well as a variety of colorful vegetables. Clara discovered the advantages of adding healthy fats, such as avocados and olive oil, to aid in nutritional absorption.

Snacking became an important part of Clara's daily routine, with nuts, seeds, and yogurt providing satisfying and nutritional options. The No Gallbladder Diet Cookbook supplied her with innovative snack options that not only delighted her taste buds but also improved her digestive health.

Clara got excellent at adapting her favorite dishes to meet her dietary requirements as she studied the cookbook's numerous recipes. She also realized the necessity of staying hydrated to aid digestion in addition to the culinary side. She made water her regular companion, infusing it with cool slices of lemon or cucumber to offer a touch of flavor without jeopardizing her health-consciousness.

Clara's routine included regular physical activity, which aided digestion and overall well-being. Clara welcomed activity as a supplement to her nutritional choices, whether it was a brisk morning stroll or an evening yoga practice.

Clara's strict commitment to her food and lifestyle paid off over time. She not only kept her health but thrived in the absence of her gallbladder. The No Gallbladder Diet Cookbook had evolved into more than just a collection of recipes; it had become a trusted companion on Clara's path to wellness.

Clara's story serves as an encouragement to those experiencing similar issues, demonstrating that a meaningful and healthy life is possible even after gallbladder removal with determination, informed choices, and the correct resources.

Welcome to the No Gallbladder Diet Cookbook, a culinary guide created to assist those living without a gallbladder. Whether you've had gallbladder surgery or are simply looking for digestive harmony, this cookbook provides a mix of delectable recipes designed to ease the transition to a gallbladder-friendly lifestyle. From savory meals that use low-fat alternatives to creative culinary solutions that prioritize digestive comfort, travel on a delectable journey meant to make every meal delightful and healthy. Discover a wealth of dishes that cater to the specific nutritional requirements of a gallbladder-free lifestyle, ensuring a delightful and nourishing culinary experience.

"My body adapts gracefully to life without a gallbladder."

"I nourish my body with foods that support digestion and overall well-being."

CHAPTER 1: EVERYTHING YOU NEED TO KNOW ABOUT GALLBLADDER

The gallbladder is a tiny organ that stores bile that the liver produces. It secretes bile into the small intestine to facilitate digestion, particularly fat breakdown.

THE IMPORTANCE OF THE GALLBLADDER

The gallbladder is an important part of the digestive system because it stores and releases bile, which aids in fat digestion. Bile aids in the emulsification of fats, making them more accessible to digestive enzymes. This mechanism is required for fat-soluble vitamin and nutrient absorption. While the gallbladder is not essential in and of itself, its function plays an important role in the human body's digestion and nutritional absorption.

WHAT ARE THE SYMPTOMS OF GALLBLADDER PROBLEM

Symptoms of gallbladder problems include:

1. Pain: Consistent pain in the upper right abdomen or under the rib cage, usually after eating.

2. Nausea and Vomiting: Feeling nauseous and maybe vomiting, especially after consuming fatty or greasy foods.

3. Indigestion: Trouble digesting fats, resulting in bloating, gas, and discomfort.

4. Jaundice: Yellowing of the skin and eyes caused by an excess of bilirubin in the bloodstream.

5. Fever and chills: Fever and chills can be caused by gallbladder inflammation or infection.

6. Stool Color Changes: Light-colored or pale feces may suggest a problem with bile flow.

7. Back Pain: Gallbladder disorders can cause pain between the shoulder blades.

WHY IT'S NECESSARY TO REMOVE THE GALLBLADDER IF IT CAUSES PROBLEM

Gallbladder removal, or cholecystectomy, is frequently advised if the gallbladder is causing persistent problems, most usually owing to gallstones or inflammation.

The necessity arises when:

1. Gallstones: If gallstones cause recurring discomfort, inflammation, or bile duct blockage, they may need to be removed to relieve symptoms.

2. Inflammation: Chronic gallbladder inflammation (cholecystitis) can cause problems and require surgical intervention.

3. Infections: Severe gallbladder infections can be fatal, and removal is required to avoid further complications.

LIFE AFTER GALLBLADDER REMOVAL

Life following gallbladder removal, also known as cholecystectomy, is usually normal, however certain changes may be required.

Here are some common factors to consider:

1. Changes in Diet: In the absence of a gallbladder, bile is discharged directly into the small intestine, which might impair fat digestion. Reintroducing fats gradually and using healthier fats may assist control stomach issues.

2. Meal Planning: Eating smaller, more frequent meals can help with digestion. Large, high-fat meals should be avoided to avoid discomfort.

3. Digestive Symptoms: Some people may first experience minor diarrhea or changes in bowel habits. As the body adjusts to the absence of the gallbladder, these symptoms usually improve.

4. Hydration: Staying hydrated is vital, especially if you're eating more fiber, because it helps avoid constipation.

5. Exercise: Regular physical activity promotes overall digestive health and can help you maintain a healthy weight.

6. Follow-up Care: It is critical to have regular check-ups with a healthcare practitioner to evaluate recovery and treat any concerns or persistent symptoms.

IMPORTANCE OF A SPECIALIZED DIET

A tailored diet is required after gallbladder removal to accommodate the alterations in digestion and fat absorption. The No Gallbladder Diet Cookbook is helpful in navigating this dietary adjustment.

Here's why a specialized diet is necessary, and how a cookbook like this will help:

1. Fat digestion: In the absence of a gallbladder, bile is continuously but slowly released into the small intestine. This can make fat digestion difficult. A tailored diet assists individuals in selecting the appropriate fats and portion amounts to avoid pain and digestive disorders.

2. Avoiding Discomfort: Certain foods, particularly those heavy in fat or greasy, might cause discomfort in those who do not have a gallbladder. The cookbook helps people choose foods that are simpler to digest, lowering the chance of post-meal pain.

3. Nutrient Absorption: The gallbladder aids in the absorption of fat-soluble vitamins (A, D, E, and K) by storing and concentrating bile. Including foods high in these vitamins in the diet helps optimum nutrient absorption.

4. Balanced Nutrition: A specialized diet focuses on consuming a variety of carbohydrates, proteins, and fats. The cookbook includes dishes that are not only appropriate for those who do not have a gallbladder, but also assure a well-balanced and nutritious diet.

5. Meal Planning: The cookbook supports people in planning easy-to-digest meals, preventing problems such as indigestion, gas, and bloating. This involves suggesting smaller, more frequent meals to help the body's modified digestion process.

6. Preventing Dietary Triggers: Certain meals might cause digestive discomfort in those who do not have a gallbladder. The cookbook assists in identifying and avoiding these triggers, resulting in a more pleasant post-surgery experience.

7. Symptom Management: Following gallbladder removal, some people may have symptoms such as diarrhea or changes in bowel habits. The cookbook tackles these concerns by offering meals that promote intestinal health.

FOODS TO AVOID AND FOODS TO EAT

Following a No Gallbladder Diet Cookbook is vital in maintaining a healthy and pleasant lifestyle after gallbladder removal.

Here's a comprehensive list of foods to eat and foods to avoid:

FOODS TO EAT

1. Lean Proteins: Choose skinless poultry, fish, lean cuts of meat, eggs, and plant-based proteins such as beans and lentils. These are easier to digest and do not strain the digestive system.

2. Healthy Fats: Include moderate amounts of healthy fats such as olive oil, avocados, and almonds. When compared to saturated or trans fats, these fats are less likely to cause stomach pain.

3. Fruits and veggies: Eat a variety of fruits and vegetables since they include important vitamins, minerals, and fiber. Start with well-cooked or peeled alternatives, as raw and fibrous kinds may be difficult to stomach at first.

4. Whole Grains: For a good source of fiber without overpowering the digestive system, choose whole grains such as brown rice, quinoa, and oats.

5. Low-Fat Dairy Products: Choose low-fat or fat-free dairy products such as yogurt and milk. Lactose-free foods may be simpler to tolerate for certain people.

6. Hydration: Stay hydrated by drinking plenty of water throughout the day. Adequate water aids digestion and prevents constipation.

7. Smaller, More Frequent Meals: Instead of three substantial meals per day, consider eating smaller, more frequent meals to assist digestion and avoid overloading the system.

FOODS TO AVOID

1. High-Fat Foods: Avoid high-fat and greasy foods because they can be difficult to digest without the gallbladder's focused bile production. Fried dishes, fatty cuts of meat, and rich desserts are examples of this.

2. Processed Foods: Processed foods should be avoided since they may include hidden fats, additives, or preservatives that might cause digestive difficulties.

3. Spicy Foods: Some people may discover that spicy foods cause digestive pain. It is best to minimize or avoid these until tolerance has been established.

4. Raw Vegetables: Raw vegetables might be difficult to stomach at first. To make them more digestible, consider boiling or peeling them.

5. High-Lactose Dairy: For those who are lactose intolerant, limit or avoid high-lactose dairy products. If lactose-free alternatives are required, use them.

6. Caffeine and alcohol: These substances can irritate the digestive system at times. Depending on individual tolerance, moderation or avoidance may be advantageous.

7. Large Meals: Avoid eating huge meals because they can tax the digestive system. Smaller, more balanced meals are easier to digest.

IMPORTANCE OF HYDRATION

Staying hydrated is important in order to live a healthy life after gallbladder removal.

Here's a full explanation of why hydration is critical:

1. Compensating for Bile Deficiency: The gallbladder stores and concentrates bile produced by the liver, assisting in fat digestion. Bile is continuously discharged into the small intestine in the absence of a gallbladder. Staying hydrated compensates for the lack of concentrated bile secreted after meals, contributing in the emulsification and digestion of lipids.

2. Preventing Constipation: Dehydration can cause constipation, which is a typical problem for those who have had their gallbladder removed. Adequate fluid consumption promotes digestive health by promoting regular bowel movements, reducing constipation, and preventing constipation.

3. Supporting Nutrient Absorption: Hydration is required for the absorption of water-soluble vitamins and minerals, which are essential for overall health. Because the gallbladder is involved in fat-soluble vitamin absorption, maintaining sufficient hydration becomes even more important after surgery.

4. Reduced Gallstone Chance: Staying hydrated may help minimize the chance of gallstone formation. Gallstones can still form in the bile ducts, and hydration promotes bile flow, reducing the chance of stone development.

5. Aiding Digestion: Proper hydration aids digestion by aiding in the breakdown of food particles and the flow of nutrients through the digestive tract. This is especially useful for people who are transitioning to a new digestive pattern following gallbladder removal.

6. Weight control: Staying hydrated can help with weight control by increasing fullness and decreasing the likelihood of overeating. This is especially important because dietary changes are required following gallbladder removal.

7. How to Avoid Dehydration-Related Symptoms: Dehydration can cause fatigue, dizziness, and headaches, among other symptoms. Individuals can alleviate these symptoms and maintain overall well-being by staying hydrated.

8. Supporting Overall Health: Hydration is essential for overall health, influencing a variety of biological functions such as temperature control, joint lubrication, and circulation. It is essential for the physiological activities of the organism.

"Every meal I prepare is a step towards a healthier, gallbladder-friendly lifestyle."

CHAPTER 2: BREAKFAST RECIPES

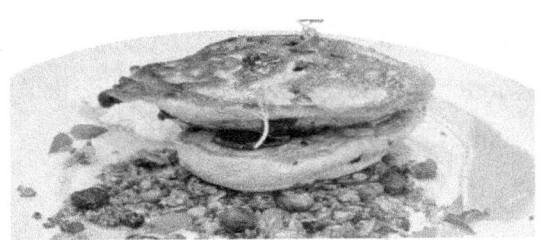

Whole Wheat Blueberry Pancakes

Ingredients:

- 1 cup whole wheat flour
- 1 tablespoon sugar
- 1 teaspoon baking powder
- 1/2 teaspoon baking soda
- 1/4 teaspoon salt
- 1 cup buttermilk
- 1 large egg
- 2 tablespoons unsalted butter, melted
- 1 cup fresh or frozen blueberries

Instructions:

1. In a large mixing bowl, whisk together the whole wheat flour, sugar, baking powder, baking soda, and salt.

2. In a separate bowl, beat the egg and then add the buttermilk and melted butter. Mix well.

3. Pour the wet ingredients into the dry ingredients and stir until just combined. Be careful not to overmix; it's okay if there are a few lumps.

4. Gently fold in the blueberries, distributing them evenly throughout the batter.

5. Heat a griddle or non-stick skillet over medium heat. Lightly grease with cooking spray or a small amount of butter.

6. Pour 1/4 cup portions of batter onto the griddle for each pancake. Cook until bubbles form on the surface, then flip and cook the other side until golden brown.

7. Repeat the process until all the batter is used, adjusting the heat if necessary to prevent burning.

8. Serve the whole wheat blueberry pancakes warm with your favorite toppings, such as maple syrup, yogurt, or additional fresh berries.

Banana Cauliflower Smoothie

Ingredients:

- 1 ripe banana
- 1 cup cauliflower florets (steamed and cooled)
- 1/2 cup plain Greek yogurt
- 1/2 cup milk (dairy or plant-based)
- 1 tablespoon honey or maple syrup (optional, depending on sweetness preference)
- 1/2 teaspoon vanilla extract
- Ice cubes (optional)

Instructions:

1. Peel the ripe banana and place it in a blender.
2. Steam the cauliflower florets until they are tender, then let them cool to room temperature.
3. Add the cooled cauliflower florets to the blender with the banana.
4. Spoon in the Greek yogurt, pour in the milk, and add the honey or maple syrup if desired.
5. Include the vanilla extract to enhance the flavor of the smoothie.
6. If you prefer a colder smoothie, you can add a handful of ice cubes to the blender.

7. Blend all the ingredients until smooth and creamy. If the smoothie is too thick, you can add more milk to achieve your desired consistency.

8. Taste the smoothie and adjust sweetness if needed by adding more honey or maple syrup.

9. Pour the banana cauliflower smoothie into glasses and serve immediately.

Buckwheat pancakes with mixed berries and a side of Greek yogurt

Ingredients:

For Buckwheat Pancakes:

- 1 cup buckwheat flour
- 1 tablespoon sugar
- 1 teaspoon baking powder
- 1/2 teaspoon baking soda
- 1/4 teaspoon salt
- 1 cup buttermilk
- 1 large egg
- 2 tablespoons unsalted butter, melted
- Cooking spray or butter for greasing the pan

For Mixed Berry Topping:

- 1 cup mixed berries (strawberries, blueberries, raspberries)

- 2 tablespoons maple syrup

For Greek Yogurt Side:

- 1 cup Greek yogurt
- 1 tablespoon honey
- 1/2 teaspoon vanilla extract

Instructions:

1. In a large bowl, whisk together the buckwheat flour, sugar, baking powder, baking soda, and salt.

2. In a separate bowl, beat the egg and then add buttermilk and melted butter. Mix well.

3. Pour the wet ingredients into the dry ingredients and stir until just combined. Be careful not to overmix; it's okay if there are a few lumps.

4. Heat a griddle or non-stick skillet over medium heat. Lightly grease with cooking spray or a small amount of butter.

5. Pour 1/4 cup portions of batter onto the griddle for each pancake. Cook until bubbles form on the surface, then flip and cook the other side until golden brown.

6. While the pancakes are cooking, prepare the mixed berry topping. In a small saucepan, combine the mixed berries and maple syrup.

Cook over medium heat for a few minutes until the berries release their juices and the syrup thickens slightly.

7. In a separate bowl, mix Greek yogurt with honey and vanilla extract to prepare the side.

8. Serve the buckwheat pancakes warm, topped with the mixed berry compote, and with a side of Greek yogurt.

Blackberry Lemon Breakfast Quinoa

Ingredients:

- 1 cup quinoa, rinsed
- 2 cups water
- 1 cup blackberries
- Zest of 1 lemon
- 2 tablespoons lemon juice
- 2 tablespoons honey
- 1/4 cup chopped nuts (e.g., almonds or walnuts)
- 1/4 cup milk (dairy or plant-based)

Instructions:

1. Rinse the quinoa under cold water thoroughly.

2. In a medium saucepan, combine the rinsed quinoa and water.

3. Bring to a boil, then reduce the heat to low, cover, and simmer for about 15 minutes or until the quinoa is cooked and the water is absorbed.

4. While the quinoa is cooking, prepare the blackberry lemon topping. In a small saucepan, combine the blackberries, lemon zest, lemon juice, and honey. Cook over medium heat for about 5 minutes, stirring occasionally, until the blackberries break down slightly and the mixture thickens. Remove from heat.

5. Once the quinoa is cooked, fluff it with a fork and transfer it to serving bowls.

6. Spoon the blackberry lemon mixture over the cooked quinoa.

7. Drizzle a bit of milk over each serving for added creaminess.

8. Sprinkle chopped nuts on top for crunch and extra flavor.

9. Serve the blackberry lemon breakfast quinoa warm and enjoy a nutritious and flavorful breakfast.

Smoothie with spinach, banana, chia seeds, and a scoop of protein powder

Ingredients:

- 1 cup fresh spinach leaves
- 1 ripe banana
- 1 tablespoon chia seeds
- 1 scoop protein powder (vanilla or your preferred flavor)
- 1 cup milk (dairy or plant-based)
- Ice cubes (optional)

Instructions:

1. Place the fresh spinach leaves in the blender.
2. Peel the ripe banana and add it to the blender.
3. Spoon in the chia seeds.
4. Add the protein powder to the blender. Choose a protein powder that complements the flavors well, such as vanilla for a sweet touch.
5. Pour in the milk of your choice.
6. If you prefer a colder smoothie, you can add a handful of ice cubes to the blender.
7. Blend all the ingredients until smooth and creamy. If the smoothie is too thick, you can add more milk to reach your desired consistency.

8. Taste the smoothie and adjust the sweetness or thickness by adding more banana, chia seeds, or milk as needed.

9. Pour the spinach, banana, chia seeds, and protein powder smoothie into a glass and enjoy your nutrient-packed and protein-rich beverage.

Healthy Coconut Yogurt with Acai Berry Granola

Ingredients:

For Healthy Coconut Yogurt:

- 2 cups unsweetened coconut yogurt
- 2 tablespoons honey or maple syrup
- 1 teaspoon vanilla extract
- 1/4 cup shredded coconut (optional, for garnish)

For Acai Berry Granola:

- 1 cup rolled oats
- 1/2 cup chopped nuts (e.g., almonds or walnuts)
- 1/4 cup coconut flakes
- 2 tablespoons chia seeds
- 2 tablespoons coconut oil, melted
- 2 tablespoons honey or maple syrup
- 1 teaspoon vanilla extract

- 1/2 cup dried acai berries (or mixed dried berries)

Instructions:

For Healthy Coconut Yogurt:

1. In a bowl, combine the unsweetened coconut yogurt, honey or maple syrup, and vanilla extract. Mix well.
2. Taste the yogurt mixture and adjust sweetness if necessary.
3. Refrigerate the coconut yogurt for at least 30 minutes to allow the flavors to meld.
4. Before serving, stir the yogurt and garnish with shredded coconut if desired.

For Acai Berry Granola:

1. Preheat the oven to 325°F (163°C).
2. In a large mixing bowl, combine rolled oats, chopped nuts, coconut flakes, and chia seeds.
3. In a separate bowl, whisk together melted coconut oil, honey or maple syrup, and vanilla extract.
4. Pour the wet mixture over the dry ingredients and toss until evenly coated.
5. Spread the granola mixture onto a baking sheet lined with parchment paper.

6. Bake for 20-25 minutes, stirring halfway through, or until the granola is golden brown and crisp.

7. Allow the granola to cool completely. Once cooled, mix in the dried acai berries or your choice of mixed dried berries.

8. Store the acai berry granola in an airtight container.

To serve:

1. Spoon the healthy coconut yogurt into bowls.

2. Top the yogurt with a generous serving of acai berry granola.

3. Optional: Drizzle with additional honey or maple syrup for extra sweetness.

Overnight oats with sliced banana and a sprinkle of flaxseeds

Ingredients:

- 1/2 cup rolled oats
- 1/2 cup milk (dairy or plant-based)
- 1/2 cup Greek yogurt
- 1 tablespoon honey or maple syrup (optional, for sweetness)
- 1 ripe banana, sliced

- 1 tablespoon ground flaxseeds

Instructions:

1. In a jar or airtight container, combine the rolled oats, milk, Greek yogurt, and honey or maple syrup if using.

2. Stir the ingredients until well combined. Ensure that the oats are fully submerged in the liquid.

3. Gently fold in the sliced banana into the oat mixture.

4. Seal the jar or container and refrigerate overnight, or for at least 4 hours, to allow the oats to absorb the liquid and soften.

5. Before serving, give the overnight oats a good stir. If the mixture is too thick, you can add a splash of milk to reach your desired consistency.

6. Sprinkle ground flaxseeds over the top of the overnight oats for added nutritional benefits.

7. Optionally, you can garnish with additional banana slices or other fruits of your choice.

8. Enjoy your convenient and nutritious overnight oats with sliced banana and flaxseeds.

Whole grain cereal with sliced peaches and low-fat milk

Ingredients:

- 1 cup whole grain cereal (such as oats, barley, or a multi-grain blend)
- 1 cup low-fat milk (dairy or plant-based)
- 2 ripe peaches, sliced
- 1 tablespoon honey or maple syrup (optional, for sweetness)
- Chopped nuts or seeds for garnish (optional)

Instructions:

1. Measure one cup of your preferred whole grain cereal and place it in a bowl.
2. Pour one cup of low-fat milk over the whole grain cereal. Adjust the amount of milk to your preferred consistency.
3. If you desire added sweetness, drizzle honey or maple syrup over the cereal and milk. Stir to combine.
4. Wash and slice the ripe peaches.
5. Arrange the sliced peaches on top of the cereal and milk mixture.
6. Optionally, sprinkle chopped nuts or seeds on the top for added texture and nutritional value.

7. Allow the cereal to soak for a minute or two to let the flavors meld.

8. Grab a spoon and enjoy your wholesome breakfast of whole grain cereal with sliced peaches and low-fat milk.

Coconut Buckwheat Pancakes

Ingredients:

- 1 cup buckwheat flour
- 1/2 cup all-purpose flour
- 2 teaspoons baking powder
- 1/2 teaspoon baking soda
- 1/4 teaspoon salt
- 1 cup coconut milk
- 2 large eggs
- 2 tablespoons coconut oil, melted
- 2 tablespoons honey or maple syrup
- 1 teaspoon vanilla extract
- Shredded coconut for garnish (optional)

Instructions:

1. In a large mixing bowl, whisk together the buckwheat flour, all-purpose flour, baking powder, baking soda, and salt.

2. In a separate bowl, whisk together the coconut milk, eggs, melted coconut oil, honey or maple syrup, and vanilla extract.

3. Pour the wet ingredients into the dry ingredients and stir until just combined. The batter may be slightly lumpy, but avoid overmixing.

4. Allow the batter to rest for about 5 minutes to let the buckwheat flour absorb the liquids.

5. Heat a griddle or non-stick skillet over medium heat. Lightly grease with coconut oil or cooking spray.

6. Pour 1/4 cup portions of batter onto the griddle for each pancake. Cook until bubbles form on the surface, then flip and cook the other side until golden brown.

7. Optional: Sprinkle shredded coconut on top of the pancakes just before flipping for added texture.

8. Repeat the process until all the batter is used, adjusting the heat if necessary to prevent burning.

9. Serve the coconut buckwheat pancakes warm with your favorite toppings, such as fresh fruit, maple syrup, or additional shredded coconut.

Whole grain bagel with smoked salmon, cream cheese, and sliced tomatoes

Ingredients:

- 1 whole grain bagel
- 4 ounces smoked salmon
- 2 tablespoons cream cheese
- 1 medium-sized tomato, thinly sliced
- Red onion, thinly sliced (optional)
- Capers for garnish (optional)
- Fresh dill for garnish (optional)
- Lemon wedges for serving

Instructions:

1. Preheat your oven to 350°F (175°C).
2. Slice the whole grain bagel in half and place the halves on a baking sheet.
3. Toast the bagel halves in the oven for about 5 minutes, or until they are lightly crispy. You can also toast them in a toaster if preferred.
4. While the bagel is toasting, spread a generous layer of cream cheese on each bagel half.

5. Arrange smoked salmon on top of the cream cheese. Ensure an even distribution across both bagel halves.

6. Place thinly sliced tomatoes on the smoked salmon. If you like, add thinly sliced red onions for an extra kick.

7. Optional: Sprinkle capers on top for a briny flavor and garnish with fresh dill for added freshness.

8. Serve the whole grain bagel with smoked salmon, cream cheese, and sliced tomatoes immediately.

9. Optionally, accompany the bagel with lemon wedges on the side for a burst of citrus flavor.

Scrambled eggs with spinach and whole grain toast

Ingredients:

- 3 large eggs
- 1 cup fresh spinach leaves, washed and chopped
- Salt and pepper to taste
- 1 tablespoon butter or olive oil
- 2 slices whole grain bread

Instructions:

1. Crack the eggs into a bowl, season with salt and pepper, and whisk until well beaten.

2. Heat the butter or olive oil in a non-stick skillet over medium heat.

3. Add the chopped spinach to the skillet and sauté for 1-2 minutes until it wilts.

4. Pour the beaten eggs over the spinach in the skillet.

5. Allow the eggs to sit undisturbed for a moment, then gently stir with a spatula, lifting and folding the eggs until they are mostly set but still slightly runny.

6. Continue to cook, stirring occasionally, until the eggs are fully cooked but still moist.

7. Toast the slices of whole grain bread until they reach your desired level of crispiness.

8. Plate the scrambled eggs alongside the whole grain toast.

9. Optionally, garnish with additional salt, pepper, or herbs of your choice.

Pineapple Onion Omelet

Ingredients:

- 3 large eggs
- 1/2 cup fresh pineapple, diced
- 1/4 cup red onion, finely chopped
- Salt and pepper to taste
- 1 tablespoon butter or olive oil
- Optional: Fresh cilantro or parsley for garnish

Instructions:

1. Crack the eggs into a bowl, season with salt and pepper, and whisk until well beaten.
2. Heat the butter or olive oil in a non-stick skillet over medium heat.
3. Add the finely chopped red onion to the skillet and sauté for 1-2 minutes until it becomes translucent.
4. Add the diced pineapple to the skillet and cook for an additional 1-2 minutes, allowing the pineapple to caramelize slightly.
5. Pour the beaten eggs over the pineapple and onion in the skillet.
6. Allow the eggs to set for a moment, then gently stir with a spatula, lifting and folding the eggs until they are fully cooked but still moist.

7. Ensure that the pineapple and onion are evenly distributed throughout the omelet.

8. Once the eggs are cooked to your liking, carefully fold the omelet in half with the spatula.

9. Transfer the pineapple onion omelet to a plate and garnish with fresh cilantro or parsley if desired.

Olive Oil and Sesame Asparagus

Ingredients:

- 1 bunch fresh asparagus, woody ends trimmed
- 2 tablespoons olive oil
- 1 tablespoon sesame oil
- 2 cloves garlic, minced
- 1 tablespoon sesame seeds
- Salt and pepper to taste
- Optional: Lemon wedges for serving

Instructions:

1. Preheat the oven to 400°F (200°C).

2. In a mixing bowl, toss the trimmed asparagus with olive oil, sesame oil, minced garlic, sesame seeds, salt, and pepper. Ensure the asparagus is evenly coated.

3. Spread the seasoned asparagus in a single layer on a baking sheet.

4. Roast the asparagus in the preheated oven for about 10-12 minutes or until they are tender but still have a slight crispiness.

5. While roasting, occasionally shake the baking sheet to ensure even cooking.

6. Once the asparagus is done, remove it from the oven and transfer it to a serving platter.

7. Optionally, squeeze fresh lemon juice over the asparagus or serve with lemon wedges on the side for a citrusy kick.

8. Garnish with additional sesame seeds if desired.

9. Serve the olive oil and sesame asparagus as a flavorful side dish to complement your meal.

Scrambled tofu with sautéed spinach and whole grain toast

Ingredients:
- 1 block firm tofu, pressed and crumbled
- 2 cups fresh spinach, washed and chopped
- 1 tablespoon olive oil
- 2 cloves garlic, minced
- 1/2 teaspoon turmeric powder (for color)

- Salt and pepper to taste
- 2 slices whole grain bread, toasted
- Optional: Nutritional yeast, sliced cherry tomatoes, or avocado for garnish

Instructions:

1. Press the firm tofu to remove excess moisture. Crumble it into small, scrambled egg-like pieces.
2. Heat olive oil in a skillet over medium heat.
3. Add minced garlic to the skillet and sauté for about 30 seconds until fragrant.
4. Add the crumbled tofu to the skillet and cook for 3-5 minutes, stirring occasionally.
5. Sprinkle turmeric powder over the tofu for color. Continue cooking for an additional 2-3 minutes.
6. Add the chopped spinach to the skillet and sauté until it wilts and combines with the scrambled tofu.
7. Season the mixture with salt and pepper to taste. Adjust the seasoning as needed.
8. Toast the whole grain bread slices until they reach your desired level of crispiness.
9. Serve the scrambled tofu and sautéed spinach mixture over the toasted whole grain bread.

10. Optional: Garnish with nutritional yeast, sliced cherry tomatoes, or avocado for added flavor and texture.

Greek yogurt smoothie with mixed berries and a tablespoon of flaxseeds

Ingredients:
- 1 cup Greek yogurt
- 1/2 cup mixed berries (strawberries, blueberries, raspberries)
- 1 tablespoon flaxseeds
- 1 tablespoon honey or maple syrup (optional, for sweetness)
- 1/2 cup milk (dairy or plant-based)
- Ice cubes (optional)

Instructions:
1. In a blender, combine the Greek yogurt, mixed berries, flaxseeds, honey or maple syrup if using, and milk.
2. If you prefer a colder smoothie, add a handful of ice cubes to the blender.
3. Blend all the ingredients until smooth and creamy. Adjust the consistency by adding more milk if needed.

4. Taste the smoothie and adjust sweetness or thickness by adding more honey or maple syrup, if desired.

5. Pour the Greek yogurt smoothie into a glass.

6. Optionally, sprinkle additional flaxseeds on top for added texture.

7. Serve the smoothie immediately and enjoy the refreshing and nutritious blend of Greek yogurt, mixed berries, and flaxseeds.

Overnight chia seed oats with pineapple and shredded coconut

Ingredients:

- 1/2 cup rolled oats
- 2 tablespoons chia seeds
- 1/2 cup coconut milk (or any milk of your choice)
- 1/2 cup pineapple chunks (fresh or canned)
- 1 tablespoon shredded coconut
- 1 tablespoon honey or maple syrup (optional, for sweetness)
- 1/2 teaspoon vanilla extract

Instructions:

1. In a jar or airtight container, combine the rolled oats, chia seeds, coconut milk, honey or maple syrup if using, and vanilla extract.

2. Stir the ingredients until well combined. Ensure that the oats and chia seeds are fully immersed in the liquid.

3. Gently fold in the pineapple chunks into the mixture.

4. Seal the jar or container and refrigerate overnight, or for at least 4 hours, to allow the oats and chia seeds to absorb the liquid and soften.

5. Before serving, give the overnight chia seed oats a good stir. If the mixture is too thick, you can add a splash of milk to reach your desired consistency.

6. Sprinkle shredded coconut on top of the oats just before serving for added texture and flavor.

7. Optionally, garnish with additional pineapple chunks and shredded coconut.

8. Enjoy this tropical-inspired overnight chia seed oats with pineapple and shredded coconut for a delicious and nutritious breakfast.

Spinach and feta omelet with whole grain toast

Ingredients:

- 3 large eggs
- 1 cup fresh spinach, washed and chopped
- 1/4 cup crumbled feta cheese
- Salt and pepper to taste
- 1 tablespoon olive oil or butter
- 2 slices whole grain bread, toasted

Instructions:

1. Crack the eggs into a bowl, season with salt and pepper, and whisk until well beaten.
2. Heat olive oil or butter in a non-stick skillet over medium heat.
3. Add the chopped fresh spinach to the skillet and sauté for 1-2 minutes until it wilts.
4. Pour the beaten eggs over the wilted spinach in the skillet.
5. Allow the eggs to set for a moment, then gently stir with a spatula, lifting and folding the eggs until they are mostly set but still slightly runny.
6. Sprinkle crumbled feta cheese evenly over one half of the omelet.

7. Carefully fold the omelet in half with the spatula, covering the feta cheese.

8. Cook for an additional minute or until the feta cheese has melted and the eggs are fully cooked but still moist.

9. Toast the slices of whole grain bread until they reach your desired level of crispiness.

10. Plate the spinach and feta omelet alongside the toasted whole grain bread.

11. Optionally, garnish with additional feta cheese or chopped fresh herbs.

Blueberry Smoothie

Ingredients:
- 1 cup blueberries (fresh or frozen)
- 1 ripe banana
- 1/2 cup Greek yogurt
- 1/2 cup milk (dairy or plant-based)
- 1 tablespoon honey or maple syrup (optional, for sweetness)
- Ice cubes (optional)

Instructions:

1. Place the blueberries, ripe banana, Greek yogurt, milk, and honey or maple syrup (if using) in a blender.
2. If you prefer a colder smoothie, add a handful of ice cubes to the blender.
3. Blend all the ingredients until smooth and creamy. Adjust the consistency by adding more milk if needed.
4. Taste the smoothie and adjust sweetness or thickness by adding more honey or maple syrup, if desired.
5. Pour the blueberry smoothie into a glass.
6. Optionally, garnish with a few whole blueberries on top for added freshness.
7. Serve the smoothie immediately and enjoy the delicious and antioxidant-rich blueberry goodness.

Quinoa Porridge

Ingredients:

- 1/2 cup quinoa, rinsed
- 1 cup milk (dairy or plant-based)
- 1/2 cup water

- 1 tablespoon honey or maple syrup
- 1/2 teaspoon vanilla extract
- Pinch of salt
- Toppings: Fresh fruit, nuts, seeds, or dried fruit (optional)

Instructions:

1. Rinse the quinoa thoroughly under cold water.
2. In a saucepan, combine the rinsed quinoa, milk, water, honey or maple syrup, vanilla extract, and a pinch of salt.
3. Bring the mixture to a boil over medium heat, then reduce the heat to low, cover, and simmer for about 15-20 minutes, or until the quinoa is cooked and the liquid is absorbed.
4. Stir occasionally to prevent sticking and ensure even cooking.
5. Once the quinoa is cooked, remove the saucepan from the heat and let it sit, covered, for a few minutes to allow the porridge to thicken.
6. Taste the quinoa porridge and adjust sweetness if needed by adding more honey or maple syrup.
7. Serve the quinoa porridge in bowls and top with your favorite toppings such as fresh fruit, nuts, seeds, or dried fruit.

8. Optionally, drizzle with a bit of additional honey or maple syrup for extra sweetness.

Oat bran muffins with blueberries and a side of low-fat yogurt

Ingredients:

- 1 cup oat bran
- 1/2 cup whole wheat flour
- 1/2 cup all-purpose flour
- 1/2 cup brown sugar, packed
- 1 teaspoon baking powder
- 1/2 teaspoon baking soda
- 1/4 teaspoon salt
- 1 cup low-fat yogurt
- 1/4 cup unsweetened applesauce
- 1/4 cup vegetable oil
- 1 large egg
- 1 teaspoon vanilla extract
- 1 cup fresh or frozen blueberries

Instructions:

1. Preheat your oven to 375°F (190°C). Line a muffin tin with paper liners or lightly grease the cups.

2. In a large bowl, combine the oat bran, whole wheat flour, all-purpose flour, brown sugar, baking powder, baking soda, and salt.

3. In a separate bowl, whisk together the low-fat yogurt, applesauce, vegetable oil, egg, and vanilla extract.

4. Pour the wet ingredients into the dry ingredients and stir until just combined. Be careful not to overmix.

5. Gently fold in the blueberries, distributing them evenly throughout the batter.

6. Spoon the batter into the prepared muffin cups, filling each about 2/3 full.

7. Bake in the preheated oven for 18-20 minutes, or until a toothpick inserted into the center of a muffin comes out clean.

8. Allow the muffins to cool in the tin for a few minutes before transferring them to a wire rack to cool completely.

9. Serve the oat bran muffins with a side of low-fat yogurt.

Smoothie bowl with mango, kiwi, and a sprinkle of pumpkin seeds

Ingredients:

For the Smoothie Base:

- 1 cup frozen mango chunks
- 1 ripe banana
- 1/2 cup Greek yogurt
- 1/2 cup almond milk (or any milk of your choice)
- 1 tablespoon honey or maple syrup (optional, for sweetness)
- Ice cubes (optional)

Toppings:

- 1 ripe kiwi, peeled and sliced
- 1 tablespoon pumpkin seeds

Instructions:

1. In a blender, combine the frozen mango chunks, ripe banana, Greek yogurt, almond milk, and honey or maple syrup if using.
2. If you prefer a thicker consistency, you can add a handful of ice cubes to the blender.
3. Blend all the ingredients until smooth and creamy. Adjust the consistency by adding more almond milk if needed.

4. Taste the smoothie and adjust sweetness if necessary by adding more honey or maple syrup.

5. Pour the smoothie into a bowl.

6. Arrange sliced kiwi on top of the smoothie base.

7. Sprinkle pumpkin seeds over the smoothie bowl for added crunch and nutritional value.

8. Optionally, drizzle a bit more honey or maple syrup over the top for extra sweetness.

9. Enjoy this vibrant and nutritious smoothie bowl with the tropical flavors of mango and kiwi, complemented by the crunch of pumpkin seeds.

Cantaloupe Smoothie

Ingredients:

- 1 cup fresh cantaloupe, cubed
- 1/2 banana
- 1/2 cup Greek yogurt
- 1/2 cup coconut water (or regular water)
- 1 tablespoon honey or maple syrup (optional, for sweetness)
- Ice cubes (optional)

Instructions:

1. In a blender, combine the fresh cantaloupe cubes, banana, Greek yogurt, coconut water, and honey or maple syrup if using.

2. If you prefer a colder smoothie, you can add a handful of ice cubes to the blender.

3. Blend all the ingredients until smooth and creamy. Adjust the consistency by adding more coconut water if needed.

4. Taste the smoothie and adjust sweetness if necessary by adding more honey or maple syrup.

5. Pour the cantaloupe smoothie into a glass.

6. Optionally, garnish with a slice of cantaloupe on the rim of the glass for a decorative touch.

7. Enjoy this refreshing and hydrating cantaloupe smoothie as a delightful drink for breakfast or a snack.

Whole grain waffles with fresh berries and a drizzle of honey

Ingredients:

- 1 cup whole wheat flour
- 1/2 cup all-purpose flour
- 2 tablespoons ground flaxseed (optional)

- 2 teaspoons baking powder
- 1/2 teaspoon baking soda
- 1/4 teaspoon salt
- 1 1/2 cups buttermilk
- 1/4 cup melted unsalted butter
- 2 tablespoons honey
- 2 large eggs
- 1 teaspoon vanilla extract

Toppings:

- Fresh berries (strawberries, blueberries, raspberries)
- Honey for drizzling

Instructions:

1. Preheat your waffle iron according to the manufacturer's instructions.
2. In a large bowl, whisk together the whole wheat flour, all-purpose flour, ground flaxseed (if using), baking powder, baking soda, and salt.
3. In a separate bowl, whisk together the buttermilk, melted butter, honey, eggs, and vanilla extract.
4. Pour the wet ingredients into the dry ingredients and stir until just combined. Be careful not to overmix; it's okay if there are a few lumps.

5. Lightly grease the waffle iron with cooking spray or a small amount of melted butter.

6. Pour the batter onto the preheated waffle iron, spreading it evenly.

7. Close the waffle iron and cook according to the manufacturer's instructions, usually for about 4-5 minutes, until the waffles are golden brown and crisp.

8. Carefully remove the waffles and repeat with the remaining batter.

9. Serve the whole grain waffles warm, topped with fresh berries, and drizzled with honey.

10. Optionally, you can garnish with additional honey or a sprinkle of flaxseeds for added flavor and nutrition.

Chocolate Chip Zucchini Muffins

Ingredients:
- 1 1/2 cups all-purpose flour
- 1/2 cup whole wheat flour
- 1 teaspoon baking powder
- 1/2 teaspoon baking soda
- 1/2 teaspoon salt
- 1 teaspoon ground cinnamon

- 1/2 cup unsalted butter, melted
- 1/2 cup granulated sugar
- 1/4 cup brown sugar, packed
- 2 large eggs
- 1 teaspoon vanilla extract
- 1 1/2 cups shredded zucchini (about 1 medium-sized zucchini)
- 1/2 cup plain Greek yogurt
- 1 cup chocolate chips (semi-sweet or dark)

Instructions:

1. Preheat your oven to 350°F (175°C). Line a muffin tin with paper liners or lightly grease the cups.

2. In a large bowl, whisk together the all-purpose flour, whole wheat flour, baking powder, baking soda, salt, and ground cinnamon.

3. In another bowl, combine the melted butter, granulated sugar, brown sugar, eggs, and vanilla extract. Mix until well combined.

4. Add the shredded zucchini to the wet ingredients and stir until evenly distributed.

5. Gradually add the dry ingredients to the wet ingredients, mixing until just combined.

6. Fold in the plain Greek yogurt until the batter is smooth.

7. Gently fold in the chocolate chips.

8. Spoon the batter into the prepared muffin cups, filling each about 2/3 full.

9. Bake in the preheated oven for 18-20 minutes, or until a toothpick inserted into the center of a muffin comes out clean.

10. Allow the muffins to cool in the tin for a few minutes before transferring them to a wire rack to cool completely.

11. Enjoy these delicious chocolate chip zucchini muffins as a delightful treat or snack!

Whole grain toast with avocado slices and a fruit salad

Ingredients:

For Whole Grain Toast with Avocado:

- 2 slices whole grain bread
- 1 ripe avocado, sliced
- Salt and pepper to taste
- Optional: Red pepper flakes or lemon juice for added flavor

For Fruit Salad:

- 1 cup mixed fresh fruit (such as berries, kiwi, grapes, and melon)
- 1 tablespoon honey or maple syrup (optional, for sweetness)
- Fresh mint leaves for garnish (optional)

Instructions:

For Whole Grain Toast with Avocado:

1. Toast the slices of whole grain bread until they reach your desired level of crispiness.
2. While the toast is still warm, carefully spread slices of ripe avocado on top.
3. Season the avocado with salt and pepper to taste.
4. Optionally, add a sprinkle of red pepper flakes for a bit of heat or a squeeze of fresh lemon juice for added brightness.

For Fruit Salad:

1. Wash and prepare the mixed fresh fruit. Cut larger fruits into bite-sized pieces.
2. In a bowl, combine the mixed fresh fruit.
3. Optionally, drizzle honey or maple syrup over the fruit for added sweetness. Toss gently to coat.

4. Garnish the fruit salad with fresh mint leaves for a burst of flavor and freshness.

To Serve:

1. Arrange the whole grain toast with avocado slices on a plate.
2. Serve the fruit salad alongside the toast.
3. Enjoy this wholesome and balanced meal of whole grain toast with creamy avocado and a refreshing fruit salad!

Apple Cinnamon Oatmeal

Ingredients:

- 1 cup rolled oats
- 2 cups water
- 1 cup milk (dairy or plant-based)
- 1 large apple, peeled, cored, and diced
- 1-2 tablespoons maple syrup or honey
- 1 teaspoon ground cinnamon
- 1/4 teaspoon nutmeg (optional)
- Pinch of salt
- Optional toppings: Sliced almonds, chopped walnuts, raisins, or a dollop of yogurt

Instructions:

1. In a saucepan, combine the rolled oats, water, and a pinch of salt. Bring to a boil over medium heat.

2. Once boiling, reduce the heat to medium-low and simmer, stirring occasionally, for about 5 minutes or until the oats begin to absorb the water.

3. Add the diced apple to the saucepan and continue to simmer for an additional 5-7 minutes, or until the apples are tender and the oats reach your desired consistency.

4. Pour in the milk and stir to combine. Simmer for an additional 2-3 minutes, or until the oatmeal is creamy.

5. Add ground cinnamon and nutmeg (if using) to the oatmeal. Stir well to incorporate the spices.

6. Sweeten the oatmeal with maple syrup or honey. Adjust the sweetness to your liking.

7. Remove the saucepan from the heat and let the oatmeal sit for a minute to allow flavors to meld.

8. Serve the apple cinnamon oatmeal in bowls.

9. Optionally, top with sliced almonds, chopped walnuts, raisins, or a dollop of yogurt for added texture and flavor.

10. Enjoy this warm and comforting apple cinnamon oatmeal for a nutritious and delicious breakfast!

Greek yogurt parfait with granola and mixed fruit

Ingredients:
- 1 cup Greek yogurt
- 1/2 cup granola
- 1 cup mixed fresh fruit (such as berries, kiwi, banana slices)
- 1 tablespoon honey or maple syrup (optional, for sweetness)
- Optional toppings: Chia seeds, shredded coconut, or chopped nuts

Instructions:
1. In a glass or bowl, start by layering a portion of Greek yogurt at the bottom.
2. Add a layer of granola on top of the Greek yogurt.
3. Follow with a layer of mixed fresh fruit.

4. Optionally, drizzle honey or maple syrup over the fruit for added sweetness.

5. Repeat the layers until the glass or bowl is filled, finishing with a final layer of fruit on top.

6. Optionally, sprinkle chia seeds, shredded coconut, or chopped nuts on the very top for added texture and nutritional benefits.

7. Serve the Greek yogurt parfait immediately, or refrigerate until ready to eat.

8. Use a long spoon to scoop through all the layers, ensuring you get a bit of yogurt, granola, and fruit in each bite.

9. Enjoy this delicious and customizable Greek yogurt parfait as a wholesome breakfast, snack, or dessert!

Oatmeal with sliced strawberries and a dollop of low-fat yogurt

Ingredients:
- 1/2 cup rolled oats
- 1 cup water
- 1/2 cup milk (dairy or plant-based)
- Pinch of salt
- 1/2 cup fresh strawberries, hulled and sliced

- 1 tablespoon honey or maple syrup (optional, for sweetness)
- 2 tablespoons low-fat yogurt

Instructions:

1. In a saucepan, combine the rolled oats, water, milk, and a pinch of salt.
2. Bring the mixture to a boil over medium heat, stirring occasionally.
3. Once boiling, reduce the heat to medium-low and simmer, stirring occasionally, for about 5 minutes or until the oats begin to absorb the liquid and reach your desired consistency.
4. Add sliced strawberries to the saucepan and continue to simmer for an additional 2-3 minutes, allowing the strawberries to soften.
5. Optional: Sweeten the oatmeal with honey or maple syrup. Adjust the sweetness to your liking.
6. Remove the saucepan from the heat and let the oatmeal sit for a minute to allow flavors to meld.
7. Transfer the oatmeal to a bowl.
8. Top the oatmeal with a dollop of low-fat yogurt.

9. Optionally, garnish with additional sliced strawberries.

10. Enjoy this simple and delightful bowl of oatmeal with sliced strawberries and a dollop of low-fat yogurt for a nutritious breakfast!

Cheesy Pancakes

Ingredients:

- 1 cup all-purpose flour
- 2 teaspoons baking powder
- 1/2 teaspoon salt
- 1 tablespoon granulated sugar
- 1 cup milk
- 1 large egg
- 2 tablespoons unsalted butter, melted
- 1 cup shredded cheese (cheddar, mozzarella, or your preferred cheese)
- Cooking spray or additional butter for greasing the pan

Instructions:

1. In a large mixing bowl, whisk together the all-purpose flour, baking powder, salt, and sugar.

2. In a separate bowl, whisk together the milk, egg, and melted butter.

3. Pour the wet ingredients into the dry ingredients and stir until just combined. The batter may be slightly lumpy, but avoid overmixing.

4. Gently fold in the shredded cheese until evenly distributed in the batter.

5. Heat a griddle or non-stick skillet over medium heat. Lightly grease with cooking spray or butter.

6. Pour 1/4 cup portions of batter onto the griddle for each pancake. Use the back of a spoon to spread the batter into a round shape.

7. Cook until bubbles form on the surface of the pancake, then flip and cook the other side until golden brown.

8. Repeat the process until all the batter is used, adjusting the heat if necessary to prevent burning.

9. Serve the cheesy pancakes warm with your favorite toppings or additional shredded cheese.

Chia seed pudding with mango chunks and a handful of pistachios

Ingredients:

- 1/4 cup chia seeds
- 1 cup milk (dairy or plant-based)
- 1 tablespoon honey or maple syrup (optional, for sweetness)
- 1/2 teaspoon vanilla extract
- 1 ripe mango, peeled, pitted, and diced
- A handful of pistachios, shelled and chopped

Instructions:

1. In a bowl, combine the chia seeds, milk, honey or maple syrup (if using), and vanilla extract.
2. Stir the mixture well to ensure the chia seeds are evenly distributed.
3. Let the chia seed mixture sit for a few minutes, then stir again to prevent clumping.
4. Cover the bowl and refrigerate for at least 3 hours or overnight to allow the chia seeds to absorb the liquid and create a pudding-like consistency.
5. Before serving, give the chia pudding a good stir to ensure it's well mixed and smooth.

6. In serving glasses or bowls, layer the chia seed pudding with diced mango chunks.

7. Sprinkle chopped pistachios on top for added crunch and flavor.

8. Optionally, drizzle a bit of honey or maple syrup over the chia pudding for extra sweetness.

9. Serve the chia seed pudding with mango chunks and pistachios chilled.

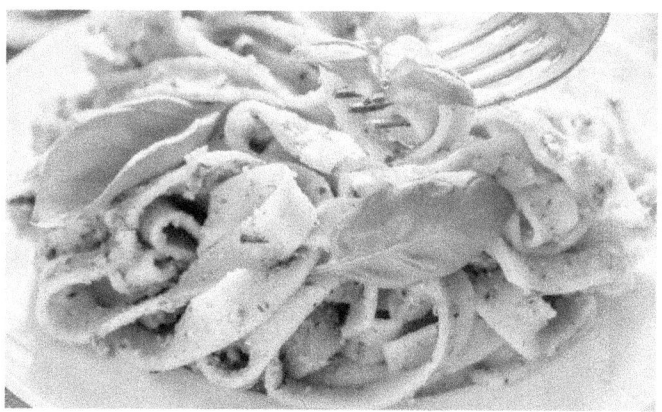

CHAPTER 3: LUNCH OPTIONS

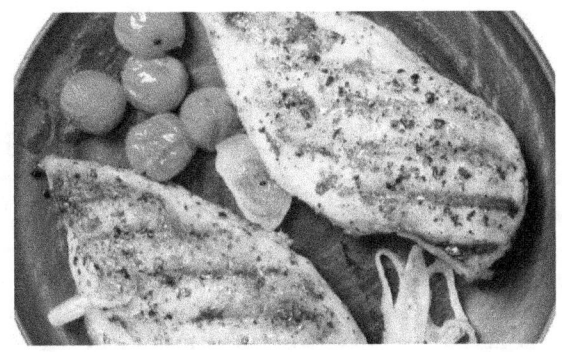

Grilled chicken breast with quinoa and steamed broccoli

Ingredients:

For Grilled Chicken Breast:

- 2 boneless, skinless chicken breasts
- 2 tablespoons olive oil
- 2 cloves garlic, minced
- 1 teaspoon dried oregano
- 1 teaspoon dried thyme
- Salt and pepper to taste
- Lemon wedges for serving (optional)

For Quinoa:

- 1 cup quinoa, rinsed
- 2 cups water or chicken broth

- Salt to taste

For Steamed Broccoli:

- 2 cups broccoli florets

Instructions:

For Grilled Chicken Breast:

1. In a bowl, mix together olive oil, minced garlic, dried oregano, dried thyme, salt, and pepper to create a marinade.

2. Place the chicken breasts in a shallow dish and coat them with the marinade. Allow them to marinate for at least 30 minutes in the refrigerator.

3. Preheat a grill or grill pan over medium-high heat.

4. Grill the chicken breasts for about 6-8 minutes per side, or until they reach an internal temperature of 165°F (74°C) and have nice grill marks.

5. Once cooked, let the chicken rest for a few minutes before slicing.

6. Optionally, serve the grilled chicken breasts with lemon wedges for added flavor.

For Quinoa:

1. In a saucepan, combine the rinsed quinoa and water or chicken broth.

2. Bring to a boil, then reduce the heat to low, cover, and simmer for about 15 minutes or until the quinoa is cooked and the liquid is absorbed.

3. Fluff the quinoa with a fork and season with salt to taste.

For Steamed Broccoli:

1. Steam the broccoli florets using a steamer basket or a microwave-safe dish with a bit of water for 3-4 minutes, or until they are tender-crisp.

2. Alternatively, you can blanch the broccoli in boiling water for 2-3 minutes.

To Serve:

1. Arrange a portion of quinoa on each plate.

2. Top the quinoa with sliced grilled chicken breasts.

3. Serve the steamed broccoli on the side or on top of the chicken.

4. Optionally, garnish with additional herbs or a drizzle of olive oil.

Turkey and vegetable stir-fry with brown rice

Ingredients:

For Turkey and Vegetable Stir-Fry:

- 1 pound ground turkey
- 2 tablespoons soy sauce (low-sodium)
- 1 tablespoon hoisin sauce
- 1 tablespoon oyster sauce
- 1 tablespoon sesame oil
- 2 tablespoons vegetable oil (divided)
- 3 cloves garlic, minced
- 1 tablespoon fresh ginger, grated
- 1 cup broccoli florets
- 1 bell pepper, thinly sliced
- 1 carrot, julienned
- 1 cup snap peas, trimmed
- Salt and pepper to taste
- Green onions for garnish (optional)
- Sesame seeds for garnish (optional)

For Brown Rice:

- 1 cup brown rice
- 2 cups water
- 1/2 teaspoon salt

Instructions:

For Brown Rice:

1. Rinse the brown rice under cold water until the water runs clear.

2. In a saucepan, combine the rinsed brown rice, water, and salt.

3. Bring to a boil, then reduce the heat to low, cover, and simmer for about 45-50 minutes or until the rice is tender and the water is absorbed.

4. Fluff the rice with a fork and let it rest, covered, for a few minutes before serving.

For Turkey and Vegetable Stir-Fry:

1. In a bowl, mix together soy sauce, hoisin sauce, and oyster sauce. Set aside.

2. Heat 1 tablespoon of vegetable oil in a large wok or skillet over medium-high heat.

3. Add the ground turkey to the wok and cook until browned, breaking it apart with a spoon as it cooks.

4. Once the turkey is browned, add minced garlic and grated ginger. Stir-fry for 1-2 minutes until fragrant.

5. Add the broccoli, bell pepper, carrot, and snap peas to the wok. Stir-fry for an additional 3-4 minutes or until the vegetables are tender-crisp.

6. Pour the sauce mixture over the turkey and vegetables. Stir well to coat everything evenly.

7. Drizzle sesame oil over the stir-fry and toss to combine.

8. Season with salt and pepper to taste.

9. Optional: Garnish the stir-fry with sliced green onions and sesame seeds.

To Serve:

1. Spoon the turkey and vegetable stir-fry over a bed of cooked brown rice.

2. Enjoy this flavorful and healthy turkey and vegetable stir-fry with brown rice!

Grilled shrimp salad with mixed greens, cherry tomatoes, and a light olive oil vinaigrette

Ingredients:

For Grilled Shrimp:

- 1 pound large shrimp, peeled and deveined
- 2 tablespoons olive oil
- 2 cloves garlic, minced
- 1 teaspoon paprika
- Salt and pepper to taste
- Lemon wedges for serving (optional)

For Salad:

- 6 cups mixed salad greens (lettuce, arugula, spinach, etc.)
- 1 cup cherry tomatoes, halved
- 1/2 red onion, thinly sliced

For Olive Oil Vinaigrette:

- 1/4 cup extra-virgin olive oil
- 2 tablespoons red wine vinegar
- 1 teaspoon Dijon mustard
- 1 teaspoon honey
- Salt and pepper to taste

Instructions:

For Grilled Shrimp:

1. In a bowl, combine olive oil, minced garlic, paprika, salt, and pepper.
2. Add the peeled and deveined shrimp to the bowl, tossing to coat them evenly with the marinade. Let them marinate for about 15-30 minutes.
3. Preheat the grill or grill pan over medium-high heat.
4. Thread the marinated shrimp onto skewers.
5. Grill the shrimp for 2-3 minutes per side, or until they are opaque and cooked through.

6. Optionally, squeeze lemon wedges over the grilled shrimp for added freshness.

For Salad:

1. In a large salad bowl, combine the mixed salad greens, cherry tomatoes, and thinly sliced red onion.

For Olive Oil Vinaigrette:

1. In a small bowl, whisk together extra-virgin olive oil, red wine vinegar, Dijon mustard, honey, salt, and pepper until well combined.
2. Adjust the seasoning to taste.

To Serve:

1. Arrange the grilled shrimp on top of the mixed greens, tomatoes, and red onion.
2. Drizzle the olive oil vinaigrette over the salad.
3. Toss the salad gently to coat the ingredients with the dressing.
4. Serve the grilled shrimp salad immediately, garnishing with additional lemon wedges if desired.

Lentil soup with a side of whole grain roll

Ingredients:

For Lentil Soup:

- 1 cup dried brown or green lentils, rinsed and drained
- 1 onion, finely chopped
- 2 carrots, diced
- 2 celery stalks, diced
- 3 cloves garlic, minced
- 1 can (14 ounces) diced tomatoes
- 6 cups vegetable or chicken broth
- 1 teaspoon ground cumin
- 1 teaspoon ground coriander
- 1 teaspoon smoked paprika
- 1/2 teaspoon ground turmeric
- Salt and pepper to taste
- 2 tablespoons olive oil
- Fresh parsley for garnish (optional)
- Lemon wedges for serving (optional)

For Whole Grain Roll:

- Store-bought whole grain rolls or homemade if preferred

Instructions:

For Lentil Soup:

1. In a large soup pot, heat olive oil over medium heat.

2. Add chopped onion, diced carrots, and diced celery. Sauté for 5-7 minutes until the vegetables are softened.

3. Add minced garlic and sauté for an additional 1-2 minutes until fragrant.

4. Stir in ground cumin, ground coriander, smoked paprika, and ground turmeric. Cook for another minute to toast the spices.

5. Pour in the rinsed lentils, diced tomatoes (with their juices), and vegetable or chicken broth.

6. Bring the soup to a boil, then reduce the heat to low, cover, and simmer for about 25-30 minutes, or until the lentils are tender.

7. Season the soup with salt and pepper to taste. Adjust the seasoning if needed.

8. Optionally, garnish the lentil soup with fresh parsley.

For Whole Grain Roll:

1. Warm the whole grain rolls according to package instructions or bake homemade rolls if using.

To Serve:

1. Ladle the warm lentil soup into bowls.
2. Serve each bowl with a side of a whole grain roll.
3. Optionally, offer lemon wedges for squeezing over the soup for added freshness.
4. Enjoy this hearty and nutritious lentil soup with a wholesome whole grain roll!

Turkey lettuce wraps with hummus and cucumber

Ingredients:

For Turkey Lettuce Wraps:

- 1 pound ground turkey
- 1 tablespoon olive oil
- 1 small onion, finely chopped
- 2 cloves garlic, minced
- 1 teaspoon ground cumin
- 1 teaspoon ground coriander
- 1/2 teaspoon chili powder

- Salt and pepper to taste
- Butter lettuce leaves (or any lettuce variety of your choice)

For Hummus and Cucumber Topping:

- 1/2 cup hummus (store-bought or homemade)
- 1 cucumber, thinly sliced

Optional Garnishes:

- Cherry tomatoes, halved
- Fresh parsley or cilantro, chopped
- Lemon wedges

Instructions:

For Turkey Lettuce Wraps:

1. In a large skillet, heat olive oil over medium heat.
2. Add finely chopped onion to the skillet and sauté for 3-4 minutes until softened.
3. Add minced garlic to the skillet and sauté for an additional 1-2 minutes until fragrant.
4. Add ground turkey to the skillet, breaking it apart with a spoon. Cook until browned.
5. Stir in ground cumin, ground coriander, chili powder, salt, and pepper. Cook for another 2-3 minutes until the spices are well incorporated and the turkey is fully cooked.

6. Remove the skillet from heat.

For Hummus and Cucumber Topping:

1. Spread a spoonful of hummus on each lettuce leaf.

2. Top with a generous portion of the cooked turkey mixture.

3. Add cucumber slices on top of the turkey.

Optional Garnishes:

1. Garnish the turkey lettuce wraps with cherry tomatoes, chopped fresh parsley or cilantro, and lemon wedges if desired.

2. Serve the turkey lettuce wraps immediately, allowing each person to customize their wraps with additional toppings.

3. Enjoy these light and flavorful turkey lettuce wraps with hummus and cucumber!

Quinoa salad with cherry tomatoes, feta cheese, and a lemon-tahini dressing

Ingredients:

For Quinoa Salad:

- 1 cup quinoa, rinsed
- 2 cups water or vegetable broth
- 1 pint cherry tomatoes, halved
- 1/2 cup crumbled feta cheese
- 1/4 cup fresh parsley, chopped
- 1/4 cup red onion, finely chopped
- 1/4 cup Kalamata olives, sliced (optional)
- Salt and pepper to taste

For Lemon-Tahini Dressing:

- 3 tablespoons tahini
- 2 tablespoons olive oil
- 2 tablespoons lemon juice
- 1 tablespoon water
- 1 clove garlic, minced
- 1 teaspoon honey or maple syrup
- Salt and pepper to taste

Instructions:

For Quinoa Salad:

1. In a medium saucepan, combine quinoa and water or vegetable broth.

2. Bring to a boil, then reduce the heat to low, cover, and simmer for about 15 minutes or until the quinoa is cooked and the liquid is absorbed.

3. Fluff the quinoa with a fork and let it cool to room temperature.

4. In a large bowl, combine the cooked quinoa, cherry tomatoes, crumbled feta cheese, chopped parsley, chopped red onion, and sliced Kalamata olives if using.

5. Season the salad with salt and pepper to taste. Toss gently to combine all the ingredients.

For Lemon-Tahini Dressing:

1. In a small bowl, whisk together tahini, olive oil, lemon juice, water, minced garlic, honey or maple syrup, salt, and pepper until smooth.

2. Taste and adjust the seasoning or consistency by adding more water if needed.

3. Pour the lemon-tahini dressing over the quinoa salad and toss to coat the salad evenly.

4. Chill the quinoa salad in the refrigerator for at least 30 minutes before serving to allow the flavors to meld.

5. Optionally, garnish with additional parsley or crumbled feta before serving.

6. Serve the quinoa salad with cherry tomatoes, feta cheese, and lemon-tahini dressing as a refreshing and nutritious side dish or a light meal.

Grilled chicken Caesar salad with cherry tomatoes and whole grain croutons

Ingredients:

For Grilled Chicken:

- 2 boneless, skinless chicken breasts
- 2 tablespoons olive oil
- 2 cloves garlic, minced
- 1 teaspoon dried oregano
- Salt and pepper to taste
- Lemon wedges for serving (optional)

For Whole Grain Croutons:

- 2 cups whole grain bread, cubed

- 2 tablespoons olive oil
- 1 teaspoon dried thyme
- Salt and pepper to taste

For Caesar Salad:

- 1 head romaine lettuce, washed and chopped
- 1 cup cherry tomatoes, halved
- 1/2 cup grated Parmesan cheese

For Caesar Dressing:

- 1/2 cup mayonnaise
- 2 tablespoons grated Parmesan cheese
- 2 tablespoons lemon juice
- 1 tablespoon Dijon mustard
- 1 clove garlic, minced
- Salt and pepper to taste

Instructions:

For Grilled Chicken:

1. In a bowl, mix together olive oil, minced garlic, dried oregano, salt, and pepper.
2. Place the chicken breasts in a shallow dish and coat them with the marinade. Let them marinate for at least 30 minutes in the refrigerator.
3. Preheat the grill or grill pan over medium-high heat.

4. Grill the chicken breasts for about 6-8 minutes per side, or until they reach an internal temperature of 165°F (74°C) and have nice grill marks.
5. Once cooked, let the chicken rest for a few minutes before slicing.
6. Optionally, serve the grilled chicken breasts with lemon wedges for added flavor.

For Whole Grain Croutons:

1. Preheat the oven to 375°F (190°C).
2. In a bowl, toss the cubed whole grain bread with olive oil, dried thyme, salt, and pepper.
3. Spread the seasoned bread cubes on a baking sheet in a single layer.
4. Bake for 10-15 minutes, or until the croutons are golden and crispy.
5. Remove from the oven and let them cool.

For Caesar Dressing:

1. In a bowl, whisk together mayonnaise, grated Parmesan cheese, lemon juice, Dijon mustard, minced garlic, salt, and pepper until well combined.
2. Adjust the seasoning to taste.

For Caesar Salad:

1. In a large salad bowl, combine chopped romaine lettuce, halved cherry tomatoes, and grated Parmesan cheese.
2. Add the sliced grilled chicken on top.
3. Drizzle the Caesar dressing over the salad and toss to coat everything evenly.
4. Add the whole grain croutons to the salad just before serving.
5. Optionally, garnish with additional grated Parmesan or a sprinkle of black pepper.
6. Serve the grilled chicken Caesar salad immediately as a delicious and satisfying meal.

Turkey and vegetable kebabs with a side of hummus and whole wheat pita

Ingredients:

For Turkey and Vegetable Kebabs:

- 1 pound ground turkey
- 1 small red onion, diced
- 1 bell pepper, diced (any color)
- 1 zucchini, sliced
- 1 tablespoon olive oil
- 2 teaspoons ground cumin

- 2 teaspoons ground coriander
- 1 teaspoon smoked paprika
- Salt and pepper to taste
- Wooden or metal skewers

For Hummus:

- 1 can (15 ounces) chickpeas, drained and rinsed
- 3 tablespoons tahini
- 2 tablespoons olive oil
- 2 tablespoons lemon juice
- 1 clove garlic, minced
- Salt to taste
- Water (as needed to achieve desired consistency)

For Whole Wheat Pita:

- Whole wheat pita bread

Instructions:

For Turkey and Vegetable Kebabs:

1. Preheat the grill or grill pan over medium-high heat.

2. In a bowl, combine ground turkey, diced red onion, diced bell pepper, sliced zucchini, olive oil, ground cumin, ground coriander, smoked paprika, salt, and pepper. Mix until well combined.

3. Take small portions of the mixture and shape them onto skewers, alternating between the turkey and vegetable pieces.

4. Grill the kebabs for about 5-7 minutes per side, or until the turkey is fully cooked and the vegetables are tender.

5. Optionally, brush the kebabs with a bit of olive oil during grilling for added flavor and moisture.

For Hummus:

1. In a food processor, combine chickpeas, tahini, olive oil, lemon juice, minced garlic, and a pinch of salt.

2. Blend until smooth, adding water as needed to achieve your desired consistency.

3. Taste and adjust the seasoning, adding more salt or lemon juice if necessary.

For Whole Wheat Pita:

1. Warm the whole wheat pita bread according to package instructions or on the grill for a minute or two.

To Serve:

1. Arrange the turkey and vegetable kebabs on a serving platter.

2. Serve with a side of hummus.

3. Optionally, serve the whole wheat pita bread alongside the kebabs and hummus.

4. Enjoy these flavorful turkey and vegetable kebabs with a side of hummus and whole wheat pita!

Chickpea and vegetable curry with quinoa

Ingredients:

For Chickpea and Vegetable Curry:

- 1 can (15 ounces) chickpeas, drained and rinsed
- 1 tablespoon coconut oil or vegetable oil
- 1 onion, finely chopped
- 2 cloves garlic, minced
- 1 tablespoon fresh ginger, grated
- 1 bell pepper, diced (any color)
- 1 zucchini, diced
- 1 carrot, diced
- 1 can (14 ounces) diced tomatoes
- 1 can (14 ounces) coconut milk
- 2 tablespoons curry powder
- 1 teaspoon ground cumin
- 1 teaspoon ground coriander
- 1/2 teaspoon turmeric

- 1/2 teaspoon chili powder (adjust to taste)
- Salt and pepper to taste
- Fresh cilantro for garnish (optional)
- Lime wedges for serving

For Quinoa:

- 1 cup quinoa, rinsed
- 2 cups water or vegetable broth
- 1/2 teaspoon salt

Instructions:

For Chickpea and Vegetable Curry:

1. In a large pot or deep skillet, heat coconut oil over medium heat.
2. Add finely chopped onion and sauté for 3-4 minutes until softened.
3. Add minced garlic and grated ginger to the pot. Sauté for an additional 1-2 minutes until fragrant.
4. Stir in curry powder, ground cumin, ground coriander, turmeric, chili powder, salt, and pepper. Cook for another minute to toast the spices.
5. Add diced bell pepper, diced zucchini, and diced carrot to the pot. Sauté for 5-7 minutes until the vegetables begin to soften.

6. Pour in diced tomatoes (with their juices), drained and rinsed chickpeas, and coconut milk. Stir well to combine.

7. Bring the curry to a simmer and let it cook for 15-20 minutes, allowing the flavors to meld and the vegetables to become tender.

8. Adjust the seasoning if needed and add more chili powder if you prefer a spicier curry.

9. Optionally, garnish the chickpea and vegetable curry with fresh cilantro before serving.

For Quinoa:

1. In a saucepan, combine quinoa, water or vegetable broth, and salt.

2. Bring to a boil, then reduce the heat to low, cover, and simmer for about 15 minutes or until the quinoa is cooked and the liquid is absorbed.

3. Fluff the quinoa with a fork.

To Serve:

1. Spoon the chickpea and vegetable curry over a bed of cooked quinoa.

2. Optionally, serve with lime wedges for squeezing over the curry.

3. Enjoy this hearty and flavorful chickpea and vegetable curry with quinoa!

Shrimp and avocado salad with mixed greens and a lime-cilantro dressing

Ingredients:

For Shrimp and Avocado Salad:

- 1 pound large shrimp, peeled and deveined
- 1 tablespoon olive oil
- 1 teaspoon paprika
- 1/2 teaspoon cumin
- Salt and pepper to taste
- 6 cups mixed salad greens (lettuce, arugula, spinach, etc.)
- 2 avocados, peeled, pitted, and sliced
- 1 cup cherry tomatoes, halved
- 1/4 cup red onion, thinly sliced
- 1/4 cup fresh cilantro, chopped
- Optional: Crumbled feta cheese or queso fresco

For Lime-Cilantro Dressing:

- 1/4 cup olive oil
- 2 tablespoons fresh lime juice
- 1 clove garlic, minced
- 1 teaspoon honey or maple syrup
- 1/4 cup fresh cilantro, chopped
- Salt and pepper to taste

Instructions:

For Shrimp:

1. In a bowl, mix together olive oil, paprika, cumin, salt, and pepper.
2. Toss the peeled and deveined shrimp in the spice mixture until evenly coated.
3. Heat a skillet over medium-high heat and cook the shrimp for 2-3 minutes per side or until they are opaque and cooked through.
4. Remove from heat and set aside.

For Lime-Cilantro Dressing:

1. In a small bowl, whisk together olive oil, fresh lime juice, minced garlic, honey or maple syrup, chopped cilantro, salt, and pepper.
2. Adjust the seasoning to taste.

For Shrimp and Avocado Salad:

1. In a large salad bowl, combine mixed salad greens, sliced avocados, halved cherry tomatoes, thinly sliced red onion, and chopped cilantro.
2. Add the cooked shrimp to the salad.
3. Drizzle the lime-cilantro dressing over the salad and toss gently to coat all ingredients.

4. Optionally, sprinkle crumbled feta cheese or queso fresco over the salad for added creaminess.

5. Serve the shrimp and avocado salad immediately as a refreshing and satisfying meal.

Quinoa-stuffed bell peppers with black beans and corn

Ingredients:

- 4 large bell peppers (any color)
- 1 cup quinoa, rinsed and drained
- 2 cups vegetable broth
- 1 can (15 oz) black beans, drained and rinsed
- 1 cup corn kernels (fresh, frozen, or canned)
- 1 cup diced tomatoes
- 1 cup shredded cheese (cheddar, Monterey Jack, or a blend)
- 1 teaspoon ground cumin
- 1 teaspoon chili powder
- 1/2 teaspoon garlic powder
- Salt and pepper to taste
- Olive oil for drizzling

Instructions:

1. Preheat your oven to 375°F (190°C).

2. Cut the tops off the bell peppers and remove the seeds and membranes. Lightly brush the outside of the peppers with olive oil and place them in a baking dish.

3. In a medium saucepan, combine the quinoa and vegetable broth. Bring to a boil, then reduce heat to low, cover, and simmer for about 15 minutes or until the quinoa is cooked and the liquid is absorbed.

4. In a large mixing bowl, combine the cooked quinoa, black beans, corn, diced tomatoes, shredded cheese, cumin, chili powder, garlic powder, salt, and pepper. Mix well to combine.

5. Spoon the quinoa mixture into each bell pepper until they are full, pressing down gently to pack the filling.

6. Top each stuffed pepper with a sprinkle of additional cheese if desired.

7. Cover the baking dish with foil and bake in the preheated oven for 25-30 minutes, or until the peppers are tender.

8. If you like, you can remove the foil during the last 5 minutes of baking to allow the cheese to melt and brown slightly.

9. Once done, remove the stuffed peppers from the oven and let them cool for a few minutes before serving.

10. Garnish with fresh cilantro, avocado slices, or a dollop of sour cream if desired.

Stir-fried shrimp with broccoli and snap peas, served over brown rice

Ingredients:

For Stir-Fried Shrimp:

- 1 pound large shrimp, peeled and deveined
- 2 tablespoons soy sauce (low-sodium)
- 1 tablespoon oyster sauce
- 1 tablespoon hoisin sauce
- 1 tablespoon cornstarch
- 1 teaspoon sesame oil
- 2 tablespoons vegetable oil (divided)
- 3 cloves garlic, minced
- 1 tablespoon fresh ginger, grated
- 1 broccoli crown, cut into florets
- 1 cup snap peas, trimmed
- 2 green onions, sliced (for garnish)

For Brown Rice:

- 1 cup brown rice

- 2 cups water
- 1/2 teaspoon salt

Instructions:

For Brown Rice:

1. Rinse the brown rice under cold water until the water runs clear.

2. In a saucepan, combine the rinsed brown rice, water, and salt.

3. Bring to a boil, then reduce the heat to low, cover, and simmer for about 45-50 minutes or until the rice is tender and the water is absorbed.

4. Fluff the rice with a fork and let it rest, covered, for a few minutes before serving.

For Stir-Fried Shrimp:

1. In a bowl, mix together soy sauce, oyster sauce, hoisin sauce, cornstarch, and sesame oil. Add peeled and deveined shrimp to the bowl, tossing to coat them evenly. Let them marinate for about 15-20 minutes.

2. Heat 1 tablespoon of vegetable oil in a wok or large skillet over medium-high heat.

3. Add minced garlic and grated ginger to the wok. Sauté for about 1-2 minutes until fragrant.

4. Add the marinated shrimp to the wok. Stir-fry for 2-3 minutes until the shrimp turn pink and opaque. Remove the shrimp from the wok and set aside.

5. In the same wok, add another tablespoon of vegetable oil.

6. Stir in broccoli florets and snap peas. Stir-fry for 3-4 minutes until the vegetables are crisp-tender.

7. Return the cooked shrimp to the wok and toss everything together to heat through.

8. Optionally, garnish the stir-fried shrimp and vegetables with sliced green onions.

To Serve:

1. Spoon the stir-fried shrimp, broccoli, and snap peas over a bed of brown rice.

2. Serve hot and enjoy this delicious and healthy stir-fried shrimp over brown rice!

Chicken and vegetable lettuce wraps with a side of sliced cucumber

Ingredients:

For Chicken and Vegetable Filling:

- 1 pound ground chicken
- 2 tablespoons soy sauce (low-sodium)

- 1 tablespoon hoisin sauce
- 1 tablespoon oyster sauce
- 1 tablespoon sesame oil
- 1 tablespoon vegetable oil
- 3 cloves garlic, minced
- 1 tablespoon fresh ginger, grated
- 1 cup water chestnuts, finely chopped
- 1 cup mushrooms, finely chopped
- 1 cup shredded carrots
- 1/4 cup green onions, sliced
- Bibb or iceberg lettuce leaves for wrapping

For Dipping Sauce:

- 3 tablespoons soy sauce (low-sodium)
- 1 tablespoon rice vinegar
- 1 teaspoon sesame oil
- 1 teaspoon honey or maple syrup
- Red pepper flakes (optional, for heat)

For Sliced Cucumber Side:

- 1 cucumber, thinly sliced

Instructions:

For Chicken and Vegetable Filling:

1. In a bowl, mix together soy sauce, hoisin sauce, and oyster sauce. Set aside.

2. Heat vegetable oil and sesame oil in a large skillet or wok over medium-high heat.

3. Add minced garlic and grated ginger to the skillet. Sauté for about 1-2 minutes until fragrant.

4. Add ground chicken to the skillet and cook until browned, breaking it apart with a spoon as it cooks.

5. Pour the sauce mixture over the cooked chicken and stir to coat evenly.

6. Add finely chopped water chestnuts, mushrooms, shredded carrots, and sliced green onions to the skillet. Stir-fry for an additional 3-5 minutes until the vegetables are tender-crisp.

7. Remove the skillet from heat.

For Dipping Sauce:

1. In a small bowl, whisk together soy sauce, rice vinegar, sesame oil, honey or maple syrup, and red pepper flakes if using. Set aside.

For Sliced Cucumber Side:

1. Thinly slice the cucumber.

To Serve:

1. Spoon the chicken and vegetable filling into individual lettuce leaves.

2. Drizzle with the dipping sauce or serve it on the side.

3. Serve the lettuce wraps with a side of thinly sliced cucumber.

4. Enjoy these delicious and light chicken and vegetable lettuce wraps with a refreshing side of cucumber!

Quinoa and kale salad with roasted chickpeas and a lemon-tahini dressing

Ingredients:

For Quinoa and Kale Salad:

- 1 cup quinoa, rinsed
- 2 cups water or vegetable broth
- 4 cups kale, destemmed and chopped
- 1 tablespoon olive oil
- Salt and pepper to taste

For Roasted Chickpeas:

- 1 can (15 ounces) chickpeas, drained and rinsed
- 1 tablespoon olive oil
- 1 teaspoon ground cumin
- 1 teaspoon smoked paprika

- Salt to taste

For Lemon-Tahini Dressing:

- 3 tablespoons tahini
- 2 tablespoons olive oil
- 2 tablespoons fresh lemon juice
- 1 clove garlic, minced
- 1 teaspoon honey or maple syrup
- Salt and pepper to taste

Optional Add-ins:

- Cherry tomatoes, halved
- Cucumber, diced
- Red onion, thinly sliced
- Avocado, sliced

Instructions:

For Quinoa and Kale Salad:

1. In a saucepan, combine quinoa and water or vegetable broth.
2. Bring to a boil, then reduce the heat to low, cover, and simmer for about 15 minutes or until the quinoa is cooked and the liquid is absorbed.
3. Fluff the quinoa with a fork and let it cool to room temperature.
4. In a large bowl, massage the chopped kale with olive oil, salt, and pepper until the leaves soften.

For Roasted Chickpeas:

1. Preheat the oven to 400°F (200°C).
2. Pat the chickpeas dry with a paper towel to remove excess moisture.
3. In a bowl, toss the chickpeas with olive oil, ground cumin, smoked paprika, and salt.
4. Spread the seasoned chickpeas on a baking sheet in a single layer.
5. Roast in the preheated oven for 25-30 minutes or until the chickpeas are crispy.

For Lemon-Tahini Dressing:

1. In a small bowl, whisk together tahini, olive oil, fresh lemon juice, minced garlic, honey or maple syrup, salt, and pepper until smooth.
2. Adjust the seasoning to taste.

To Assemble:

1. In the large bowl with massaged kale, add the cooked quinoa and roasted chickpeas.
2. If desired, add cherry tomatoes, cucumber, red onion, and avocado for additional freshness.
3. Drizzle the lemon-tahini dressing over the salad.
4. Toss everything together until well combined.

5. Serve the quinoa and kale salad immediately, or refrigerate for a while to let the flavors meld.

Baked chicken thighs with a side of barley and roasted vegetables

Ingredients:

For Baked Chicken Thighs:

- 4-6 bone-in, skin-on chicken thighs
- 2 tablespoons olive oil
- 2 teaspoons garlic powder
- 2 teaspoons onion powder
- 1 teaspoon paprika
- 1 teaspoon dried thyme
- Salt and pepper to taste
- Fresh parsley for garnish (optional)

For Barley:

- 1 cup pearl barley
- 3 cups chicken broth or water
- Salt to taste

For Roasted Vegetables:

- 1 pound mixed vegetables (carrots, broccoli, bell peppers, etc.), chopped
- 2 tablespoons olive oil
- Salt and pepper to taste

- 1 teaspoon dried rosemary (optional)

Instructions:

For Baked Chicken Thighs:

1. Preheat the oven to 400°F (200°C).
2. In a small bowl, mix together garlic powder, onion powder, paprika, dried thyme, salt, and pepper.
3. Pat the chicken thighs dry with a paper towel. Rub the chicken thighs with olive oil, ensuring they are well-coated.
4. Sprinkle the spice mixture evenly over both sides of the chicken thighs.
5. Place the seasoned chicken thighs on a baking sheet lined with parchment paper or a greased baking dish, skin-side up.
6. Bake in the preheated oven for 35-45 minutes or until the chicken reaches an internal temperature of 165°F (74°C) and the skin is crispy and golden.
7. Optionally, garnish the baked chicken thighs with fresh parsley before serving.

For Barley:

1. Rinse the pearl barley under cold water.

2. In a saucepan, combine the rinsed barley, chicken broth or water, and salt.

3. Bring to a boil, then reduce the heat to low, cover, and simmer for about 40-45 minutes or until the barley is tender and the liquid is absorbed.

4. Fluff the barley with a fork.

For Roasted Vegetables:

1. Preheat the oven to 425°F (220°C).

2. In a large bowl, toss the chopped mixed vegetables with olive oil, salt, pepper, and dried rosemary if using.

3. Spread the seasoned vegetables on a baking sheet in a single layer.

4. Roast in the preheated oven for 20-25 minutes or until the vegetables are golden and tender, stirring halfway through.

To Serve:

1. Plate the baked chicken thighs alongside a serving of barley and roasted vegetables.

2. Optionally, garnish with additional fresh herbs.

3. Enjoy this wholesome and satisfying meal of baked chicken thighs with a side of barley and roasted vegetables!

Turkey and vegetable wraps with whole wheat tortillas

Ingredients:

For Turkey and Vegetable Filling:

- 1 pound ground turkey
- 1 tablespoon olive oil
- 1 small onion, finely chopped
- 1 bell pepper, thinly sliced (any color)
- 1 zucchini, thinly sliced
- 2 cloves garlic, minced
- 1 teaspoon ground cumin
- 1 teaspoon chili powder
- Salt and pepper to taste
- 1 cup cherry tomatoes, halved
- 1/4 cup fresh cilantro, chopped
- Juice of 1 lime

For Whole Wheat Tortillas:

- 6 whole wheat tortillas

Optional Toppings:

- Avocado slices
- Shredded lettuce
- Greek yogurt or sour cream

Instructions:

For Turkey and Vegetable Filling:

1. In a large skillet, heat olive oil over medium heat.

2. Add finely chopped onion to the skillet and sauté for 3-4 minutes until softened.

3. Add minced garlic to the skillet and sauté for an additional 1-2 minutes until fragrant.

4. Add ground turkey to the skillet, breaking it apart with a spoon. Cook until browned.

5. Stir in ground cumin, chili powder, salt, and pepper. Cook for another 2-3 minutes until the spices are well incorporated.

6. Add thinly sliced bell pepper and zucchini to the skillet. Sauté for 5-7 minutes until the vegetables are tender.

7. Stir in cherry tomatoes, fresh cilantro, and lime juice. Cook for an additional 2 minutes until the tomatoes are slightly softened.

8. Remove the skillet from heat.

For Whole Wheat Tortillas:

1. Warm the whole wheat tortillas in a dry skillet or microwave according to package instructions.

To Assemble:

1. Spoon the turkey and vegetable filling onto the center of each whole wheat tortilla.
2. Optionally, top with avocado slices, shredded lettuce, and a dollop of Greek yogurt or sour cream.
3. Fold the sides of the tortilla over the filling and roll it up tightly to form a wrap.
4. Serve the turkey and vegetable wraps immediately.
5. Enjoy these delicious and nutritious turkey and vegetable wraps with whole wheat tortillas!

Lentil and vegetable stir-fry with quinoa

Ingredients:

For Lentil and Vegetable Stir-Fry:

- 1 cup dry lentils, rinsed
- 2 cups water
- 2 tablespoons olive oil
- 1 onion, thinly sliced
- 2 carrots, julienned
- 1 bell pepper, thinly sliced (any color)
- 1 zucchini, thinly sliced

- 2 cloves garlic, minced
- 1 tablespoon ginger, grated
- 1 cup broccoli florets
- 1 cup snap peas, trimmed
- 1/4 cup soy sauce (low-sodium)
- 2 tablespoons hoisin sauce
- 1 tablespoon rice vinegar
- 1 teaspoon sesame oil
- Sesame seeds for garnish (optional)
- Green onions, sliced for garnish (optional)

For Quinoa:

- 1 cup quinoa, rinsed
- 2 cups water or vegetable broth
- 1/2 teaspoon salt

Instructions:

For Lentil and Vegetable Stir-Fry:

1. In a saucepan, combine rinsed lentils and water. Bring to a boil, then reduce the heat to low, cover, and simmer for about 20-25 minutes or until the lentils are tender but still hold their shape. Drain any excess water.

2. In a large skillet or wok, heat olive oil over medium-high heat.

3. Add thinly sliced onion to the skillet and sauté for 3-4 minutes until softened.

4. Stir in julienned carrots, thinly sliced bell pepper, and sliced zucchini. Sauté for an additional 5-7 minutes until the vegetables are tender-crisp.

5. Add minced garlic and grated ginger to the skillet. Sauté for 1-2 minutes until fragrant.

6. Add broccoli florets and trimmed snap peas to the skillet. Stir-fry for another 3-4 minutes until the broccoli is bright green and slightly tender.

7. Incorporate cooked lentils into the vegetable mixture.

8. In a small bowl, whisk together soy sauce, hoisin sauce, rice vinegar, and sesame oil.

9. Pour the sauce over the lentil and vegetable mixture. Stir to coat everything evenly. Cook for an additional 2-3 minutes.

10. Optionally, garnish the stir-fry with sesame seeds and sliced green onions.

For Quinoa:

1. In a separate saucepan, combine quinoa, water or vegetable broth, and salt.

2. Bring to a boil, then reduce the heat to low, cover, and simmer for about 15 minutes or until the quinoa is cooked and the liquid is absorbed.

3. Fluff the quinoa with a fork.

To Serve:

1. Spoon the lentil and vegetable stir-fry over a bed of cooked quinoa.

2. Enjoy this wholesome and flavorful lentil and vegetable stir-fry with quinoa!

Quinoa and black bean salad with corn, cherry tomatoes, and avocado

Ingredients:

For Quinoa and Black Bean Salad:

- 1 cup quinoa, rinsed
- 2 cups water or vegetable broth
- 1 can (15 ounces) black beans, drained and rinsed
- 1 cup corn kernels (fresh, frozen, or canned)
- 1 cup cherry tomatoes, halved
- 1 avocado, diced
- 1/4 cup red onion, finely chopped
- 1/4 cup fresh cilantro, chopped

For Lime-Cumin Vinaigrette:

- 3 tablespoons olive oil
- 2 tablespoons fresh lime juice
- 1 teaspoon ground cumin

- 1 clove garlic, minced
- Salt and pepper to taste

Instructions:

For Quinoa and Black Bean Salad:

1. In a saucepan, combine quinoa and water or vegetable broth.
2. Bring to a boil, then reduce the heat to low, cover, and simmer for about 15 minutes or until the quinoa is cooked and the liquid is absorbed.

3. Fluff the quinoa with a fork and let it cool to room temperature.
4. In a large bowl, combine cooked quinoa, black beans, corn kernels, cherry tomatoes, diced avocado, chopped red onion, and fresh cilantro.

For Lime-Cumin Vinaigrette:

1. In a small bowl, whisk together olive oil, fresh lime juice, ground cumin, minced garlic, salt, and pepper.
2. Adjust the seasoning to taste.

To Assemble:

1. Pour the lime-cumin vinaigrette over the quinoa and black bean salad.

2. Gently toss the salad until all ingredients are well coated with the vinaigrette.

3. Refrigerate the salad for at least 30 minutes to allow the flavors to meld.

4. Serve the quinoa and black bean salad chilled.

5. Optionally, garnish with additional fresh cilantro before serving.

6. Enjoy this refreshing and nutritious quinoa and black bean salad with corn, cherry tomatoes, and avocado!

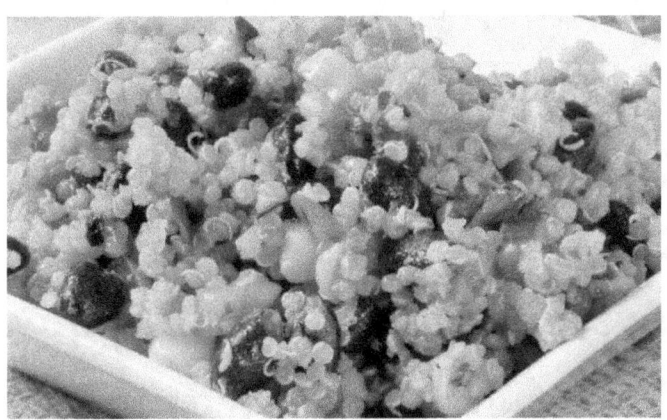

"My body is resilient, adapting effortlessly to the changes, promoting overall health and vitality."

"I choose foods that nurture my digestive system, promoting balance and harmony within."

CHAPTER 4: DINNER CREATIONS

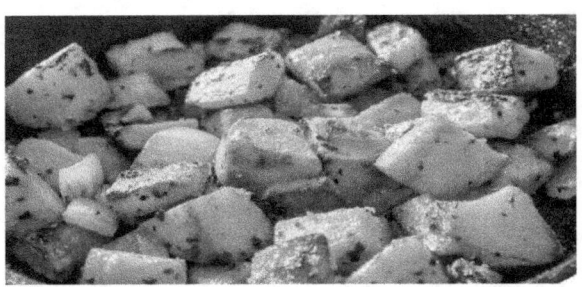

Baked fish with a side of roasted sweet potatoes and mixed vegetables

Ingredients:

For Baked Fish:

- 4 fish filets (such as cod, tilapia, or salmon)
- 2 tablespoons olive oil
- 2 tablespoons lemon juice
- 2 cloves garlic, minced
- 1 teaspoon dried oregano
- 1 teaspoon paprika
- Salt and pepper to taste
- Lemon slices for garnish

For Roasted Sweet Potatoes:

- 2 large sweet potatoes, peeled and diced
- 2 tablespoons olive oil
- 1 teaspoon dried rosemary
- Salt and pepper to taste

For Mixed Vegetables:

- 2 cups mixed vegetables (broccoli, bell peppers, cherry tomatoes, etc.), chopped
- 2 tablespoons olive oil
- 1 teaspoon dried thyme
- Salt and pepper to taste

Instructions:

For Baked Fish:

1. Preheat the oven to 400°F (200°C).
2. In a small bowl, whisk together olive oil, lemon juice, minced garlic, dried oregano, paprika, salt, and pepper.
3. Place the fish filets in a baking dish. Pour the marinade over the fish, ensuring each filet is well-coated.
4. Let the fish marinate for about 15-20 minutes.
5. Bake in the preheated oven for 15-20 minutes or until the fish is cooked through and flakes easily with a fork.

6. Optionally, garnish with lemon slices before serving.

For Roasted Sweet Potatoes:

1. In a bowl, toss diced sweet potatoes with olive oil, dried rosemary, salt, and pepper until evenly coated.

2. Spread the sweet potatoes on a baking sheet in a single layer.

3. Roast in the preheated oven for 25-30 minutes or until the sweet potatoes are tender and lightly browned, stirring halfway through.

For Mixed Vegetables:

1. In a bowl, toss chopped mixed vegetables with olive oil, dried thyme, salt, and pepper until well coated.

2. Spread the vegetables on a separate baking sheet in a single layer.

3. Roast in the preheated oven for 15-20 minutes or until the vegetables are tender-crisp, stirring halfway through.

To Serve:

1. Place a baked fish filet on each plate.

2. Serve with a side of roasted sweet potatoes and mixed vegetables.

3. Enjoy this wholesome and balanced meal of baked fish with roasted sweet potatoes and mixed vegetables!

Salmon filet with asparagus and quinoa

Ingredients:

For Salmon Filet:

- 4 salmon filets
- 2 tablespoons olive oil
- 2 tablespoons lemon juice
- 2 cloves garlic, minced
- 1 teaspoon dried dill
- Salt and pepper to taste
- Lemon slices for garnish

For Asparagus:

- 1 bunch asparagus, woody ends trimmed
- 1 tablespoon olive oil
- Salt and pepper to taste

For Quinoa:

- 1 cup quinoa, rinsed
- 2 cups water or vegetable broth
- 1/2 teaspoon salt

Instructions:

For Salmon Filet:

1. Preheat the oven to 400°F (200°C).

2. In a small bowl, whisk together olive oil, lemon juice, minced garlic, dried dill, salt, and pepper.

3. Place the salmon filets on a baking sheet. Pour the marinade over the salmon, ensuring each filet is well-coated.

4. Let the salmon marinate for about 15-20 minutes.

5. Bake in the preheated oven for 12-15 minutes or until the salmon is cooked through and flakes easily with a fork.

6. Optionally, garnish with lemon slices before serving.

For Asparagus:

1. Toss trimmed asparagus with olive oil, salt, and pepper in a bowl until evenly coated.

2. Spread the asparagus on a baking sheet in a single layer.

3. Roast in the preheated oven for 10-12 minutes or until the asparagus is tender but still crisp.

For Quinoa:

1. In a saucepan, combine rinsed quinoa, water or vegetable broth, and salt.
2. Bring to a boil, then reduce the heat to low, cover, and simmer for about 15 minutes or until the quinoa is cooked and the liquid is absorbed.
3. Fluff the quinoa with a fork.

To Serve:

1. Plate the salmon filets alongside a serving of quinoa and roasted asparagus.
2. Optionally, garnish with additional fresh dill and lemon wedges.
3. Enjoy this flavorful and nutritious meal of salmon filet with asparagus and quinoa!

Stir-fried tofu with broccoli and quinoa

Ingredients:

For Stir-Fried Tofu:

- 1 block extra-firm tofu, pressed and cubed
- 3 tablespoons soy sauce (low-sodium)
- 1 tablespoon hoisin sauce

- 1 tablespoon rice vinegar
- 1 tablespoon sesame oil
- 1 tablespoon cornstarch
- 2 tablespoons vegetable oil (for frying)
- 2 cloves garlic, minced
- 1 tablespoon fresh ginger, grated
- Red pepper flakes (optional, for heat)

For Broccoli:

- 2 cups broccoli florets
- 1 tablespoon vegetable oil
- 2 tablespoons water
- Salt to taste

For Quinoa:

- 1 cup quinoa, rinsed
- 2 cups water or vegetable broth
- 1/2 teaspoon salt

Instructions:

For Stir-Fried Tofu:

1. In a bowl, whisk together soy sauce, hoisin sauce, rice vinegar, sesame oil, and cornstarch.
2. Toss the cubed tofu in the marinade, ensuring each piece is well-coated. Let it marinate for at least 15 minutes.

3. Heat vegetable oil in a large skillet or wok over medium-high heat.

4. Add marinated tofu cubes to the skillet, reserving the marinade. Fry the tofu for 5-7 minutes or until golden brown on all sides.

5. Remove the tofu from the skillet and set aside.

6. In the same skillet, add minced garlic, grated ginger, and red pepper flakes if using. Sauté for about 1-2 minutes until fragrant.

7. Pour the reserved marinade into the skillet. Bring it to a simmer and cook for 2-3 minutes until it thickens slightly.

8. Return the fried tofu to the skillet. Toss to coat the tofu evenly with the sauce. Cook for an additional 2-3 minutes.

For Broccoli:

1. In a separate pan, heat vegetable oil over medium-high heat.

2. Add broccoli florets to the pan. Sauté for 2-3 minutes until they start to brown.

3. Add water to the pan and cover it with a lid. Steam the broccoli for an additional 2-3 minutes until it's tender but still crisp.

4. Season the broccoli with salt to taste.

For Quinoa:

1. In a saucepan, combine rinsed quinoa, water or vegetable broth, and salt.

2. Bring to a boil, then reduce the heat to low, cover, and simmer for about 15 minutes or until the quinoa is cooked and the liquid is absorbed.

3. Fluff the quinoa with a fork.

To Serve:

1. Plate the stir-fried tofu on a bed of quinoa, with a side of sautéed broccoli.

2. Optionally, garnish with sesame seeds or chopped green onions.

3. Enjoy this flavorful and protein-packed stir-fried tofu with broccoli and quinoa!

Baked chicken thighs with sweet potato wedges and green beans

Ingredients:

For Baked Chicken Thighs:

- 4-6 bone-in, skin-on chicken thighs
- 2 tablespoons olive oil
- 1 teaspoon paprika
- 1 teaspoon garlic powder
- 1 teaspoon onion powder

- 1 teaspoon dried thyme
- Salt and pepper to taste
- Fresh parsley for garnish (optional)

For Sweet Potato Wedges:

- 2 large sweet potatoes, peeled and cut into wedges
- 2 tablespoons olive oil
- 1 teaspoon smoked paprika
- 1 teaspoon cumin
- Salt and pepper to taste

For Green Beans:

- 2 cups green beans, trimmed
- 1 tablespoon olive oil
- 2 cloves garlic, minced
- Lemon zest (optional)
- Salt and pepper to taste

Instructions:

For Baked Chicken Thighs:

1. Preheat the oven to 400°F (200°C).
2. In a small bowl, mix together olive oil, paprika, garlic powder, onion powder, dried thyme, salt, and pepper.

3. Pat the chicken thighs dry with a paper towel. Rub the chicken thighs with the spice mixture, ensuring they are well-coated.

4. Place the chicken thighs on a baking sheet lined with parchment paper or a greased baking dish, skin-side up.

5. Bake in the preheated oven for 35-45 minutes or until the chicken reaches an internal temperature of 165°F (74°C) and the skin is crispy and golden.

6. Optionally, garnish with fresh parsley before serving.

For Sweet Potato Wedges:

1. In a bowl, toss sweet potato wedges with olive oil, smoked paprika, cumin, salt, and pepper until evenly coated.

2. Spread the sweet potato wedges on a baking sheet in a single layer.

3. Roast in the preheated oven for 25-30 minutes or until the sweet potato wedges are tender and lightly browned, stirring halfway through.

For Green Beans:

1. In a pan, heat olive oil over medium-high heat.

2. Add minced garlic to the pan and sauté for 1-2 minutes until fragrant.

3. Add trimmed green beans to the pan. Sauté for 5-7 minutes until the green beans are tender-crisp.

4. Optionally, sprinkle lemon zest over the green beans for added freshness.

To Serve:

1. Plate the baked chicken thighs alongside sweet potato wedges and sautéed green beans.

2. Optionally, garnish with additional fresh parsley.

3. Enjoy this wholesome and flavorful meal of baked chicken thighs with sweet potato wedges and green beans!

Grilled cod with quinoa pilaf and roasted Brussels sprouts

Ingredients:

For Grilled Cod:

- 4 cod filets
- 2 tablespoons olive oil
- 2 tablespoons lemon juice
- 2 cloves garlic, minced
- 1 teaspoon dried oregano

- Salt and pepper to taste
- Lemon wedges for serving

For Quinoa Pilaf:

- 1 cup quinoa, rinsed
- 2 cups vegetable broth
- 1 tablespoon olive oil
- 1 small onion, finely chopped
- 1 carrot, diced
- 1 celery stalk, diced
- 1/4 cup chopped parsley
- Salt and pepper to taste

For Roasted Brussels Sprouts:

- 1 pound Brussels sprouts, trimmed and halved
- 2 tablespoons olive oil
- 1 teaspoon garlic powder
- Salt and pepper to taste

Instructions:

For Grilled Cod:

1. In a bowl, whisk together olive oil, lemon juice, minced garlic, dried oregano, salt, and pepper.
2. Place the cod filets in a shallow dish. Pour the marinade over the cod, ensuring each filet is well-coated. Let it marinate for at least 15-20 minutes.

3. Preheat the grill to medium-high heat.

4. Grill the cod filets for 4-5 minutes per side or until the fish is opaque and flakes easily with a fork.

5. Optionally, serve with lemon wedges.

For Quinoa Pilaf:

1. In a saucepan, heat olive oil over medium heat.

2. Add finely chopped onion, diced carrot, and diced celery to the pan. Sauté for 3-4 minutes until the vegetables are softened.

3. Add rinsed quinoa to the pan. Stir to coat the quinoa in the vegetables and oil.

4. Pour in vegetable broth and bring to a boil. Reduce the heat to low, cover, and simmer for about 15 minutes or until the quinoa is cooked and the liquid is absorbed.

5. Fluff the quinoa with a fork and stir in chopped parsley. Season with salt and pepper to taste.

For Roasted Brussels Sprouts:

1. Preheat the oven to 400°F (200°C).

2. In a bowl, toss halved Brussels sprouts with olive oil, garlic powder, salt, and pepper until evenly coated.

3. Spread the Brussels sprouts on a baking sheet in a single layer.

4. Roast in the preheated oven for 20-25 minutes or until the Brussels sprouts are golden brown and crispy on the edges.

To Serve:

1. Plate the grilled cod on a bed of quinoa pilaf.

2. Serve with a side of roasted Brussels sprouts.

3. Enjoy this delicious and balanced meal of grilled cod with quinoa pilaf and roasted Brussels sprouts!

Baked trout with lemon and dill, served with brown rice and steamed asparagus

Ingredients:

For Baked Trout:

- 4 trout filets
- 2 tablespoons olive oil
- 2 tablespoons lemon juice
- 2 cloves garlic, minced
- 1 tablespoon fresh dill, chopped
- Salt and pepper to taste

- Lemon slices for garnish

For Brown Rice:
- 1 cup brown rice
- 2 cups water or vegetable broth
- 1/2 teaspoon salt

For Steamed Asparagus:
- 1 pound asparagus, trimmed
- 2 tablespoons olive oil
- Salt and pepper to taste

Instructions:

For Baked Trout:
1. Preheat the oven to 400°F (200°C).
2. In a bowl, whisk together olive oil, lemon juice, minced garlic, chopped fresh dill, salt, and pepper.
3. Place the trout filets on a baking sheet lined with parchment paper or a greased baking dish.
4. Brush the trout filets with the lemon-dill marinade, ensuring each filet is well-coated.
5. Optionally, place lemon slices on top of each filet.
6. Bake in the preheated oven for 12-15 minutes or until the trout is cooked through and flakes easily with a fork.

For Brown Rice:

1. In a saucepan, combine brown rice, water or vegetable broth, and salt.

2. Bring to a boil, then reduce the heat to low, cover, and simmer for about 45-50 minutes or until the brown rice is tender and the liquid is absorbed.

3. Fluff the brown rice with a fork.

For Steamed Asparagus:

1. In a steamer basket or a microwave-safe dish, place trimmed asparagus.

2. Steam in the steamer basket or microwave for 3-5 minutes or until the asparagus is tender but still crisp.

3. Drizzle olive oil over the steamed asparagus and season with salt and pepper to taste.

To Serve:

1. Plate the baked trout filets on each serving dish.

2. Serve with a side of brown rice and steamed asparagus.

3. Optionally, garnish with additional fresh dill and lemon wedges.

4. Enjoy this light and flavorful meal of baked trout with lemon and dill, served with brown rice and steamed asparagus!

Stir-fried beef with colorful bell peppers and brown rice

Ingredients:

For Stir-Fried Beef:

- 1 pound flank steak, thinly sliced
- 3 tablespoons soy sauce (low-sodium)
- 2 tablespoons oyster sauce
- 1 tablespoon hoisin sauce
- 1 tablespoon cornstarch
- 2 tablespoons vegetable oil
- 3 cloves garlic, minced
- 1 tablespoon fresh ginger, grated
- 1 red bell pepper, thinly sliced
- 1 yellow bell pepper, thinly sliced
- 1 green bell pepper, thinly sliced
- 1 onion, thinly sliced
- Green onions, sliced for garnish (optional)
- Sesame seeds for garnish (optional)

For Brown Rice:

- 1 cup brown rice

- 2 cups water
- 1/2 teaspoon salt

Instructions:

For Stir-Fried Beef:

1. In a bowl, mix together soy sauce, oyster sauce, hoisin sauce, and cornstarch to create the marinade.

2. Place the thinly sliced flank steak in the marinade, ensuring each slice is coated. Let it marinate for at least 15-20 minutes.

3. Heat vegetable oil in a wok or large skillet over high heat.

4. Add minced garlic and grated ginger to the hot oil. Sauté for about 1-2 minutes until fragrant.

5. Add the marinated flank steak to the wok. Stir-fry for 2-3 minutes or until the beef is browned and cooked through. Remove the beef from the wok and set aside.

6. In the same wok, add a bit more oil if needed. Add thinly sliced bell peppers and onion. Stir-fry for 3-4 minutes until the vegetables are tender-crisp.

7. Return the cooked beef to the wok with the vegetables. Toss to combine and heat through.

8. Optionally, garnish with sliced green onions and sesame seeds.

For Brown Rice:

1. In a saucepan, combine brown rice, water, and salt.
2. Bring to a boil, then reduce the heat to low, cover, and simmer for about 45-50 minutes or until the brown rice is tender and the liquid is absorbed.
3. Fluff the brown rice with a fork.

To Serve:

1. Plate the stir-fried beef with colorful bell peppers on each serving dish.
2. Serve with a side of brown rice.
3. Enjoy this flavorful and colorful stir-fried beef with bell peppers, served with brown rice!

Baked turkey meatballs with zucchini noodles and marinara sauce

Ingredients:

For Baked Turkey Meatballs:

- 1 pound ground turkey
- 1/2 cup breadcrumbs
- 1/4 cup grated Parmesan cheese
- 1/4 cup chopped fresh parsley
- 1 egg

- 2 cloves garlic, minced
- 1 teaspoon dried oregano
- 1/2 teaspoon dried basil
- Salt and pepper to taste

For Zucchini Noodles:

- 4 medium-sized zucchini, spiralized
- 2 tablespoons olive oil
- Salt and pepper to taste

For Marinara Sauce:

- 2 cups tomato sauce
- 1 tablespoon olive oil
- 1 onion, finely chopped
- 2 cloves garlic, minced
- 1 teaspoon dried oregano
- 1 teaspoon dried basil
- Salt and pepper to taste
- Fresh basil leaves for garnish (optional)

Instructions:

For Baked Turkey Meatballs:

1. Preheat the oven to 400°F (200°C).
2. In a large bowl, combine ground turkey, breadcrumbs, grated Parmesan cheese, chopped fresh parsley, egg, minced garlic, dried oregano, dried basil, salt, and pepper.
3. Mix the ingredients until well combined.

4. Shape the mixture into meatballs, about 1 to 1.5 inches in diameter, and place them on a baking sheet lined with parchment paper.

5. Bake in the preheated oven for 20-25 minutes or until the meatballs are cooked through and browned.

For Zucchini Noodles:

1. Spiralize the zucchini into noodles using a spiralizer.

2. Heat olive oil in a large pan over medium heat.

3. Add the zucchini noodles to the pan and sauté for 2-3 minutes until they are just tender but still have a bit of bite.

4. Season the zucchini noodles with salt and pepper to taste.

For Marinara Sauce:

1. In a saucepan, heat olive oil over medium heat.

2. Add finely chopped onion and minced garlic to the pan. Sauté for 3-4 minutes until the onion is softened.

3. Pour in the tomato sauce and add dried oregano, dried basil, salt, and pepper. Stir to combine.

4. Simmer the marinara sauce for 10-15 minutes, allowing the flavors to meld.

To Serve:

1. Plate the baked turkey meatballs on a bed of zucchini noodles.

2. Spoon marinara sauce over the meatballs and noodles.

3. Optionally, garnish with fresh basil leaves.

4. Enjoy this light and flavorful meal of baked turkey meatballs with zucchini noodles and marinara sauce!

Grilled lean pork chops with sweet potato mash and green beans

Ingredients:

For Grilled Lean Pork Chops:

- 4 lean pork chops
- 2 tablespoons olive oil
- 2 cloves garlic, minced
- 1 teaspoon dried thyme
- 1 teaspoon paprika
- Salt and pepper to taste

For Sweet Potato Mash:

- 2 large sweet potatoes, peeled and diced
- 2 tablespoons unsalted butter
- 1/4 cup milk (or more for desired consistency)

- Salt and pepper to taste

For Green Beans:
- 1 pound green beans, trimmed
- 2 tablespoons olive oil
- 2 cloves garlic, minced
- Salt and pepper to taste
- Lemon zest (optional)

Instructions:

For Grilled Lean Pork Chops:

1. Preheat the grill to medium-high heat.
2. In a bowl, mix together olive oil, minced garlic, dried thyme, paprika, salt, and pepper to create a marinade.
3. Brush the pork chops with the marinade, ensuring each chop is well-coated.
4. Grill the pork chops for 4-5 minutes per side or until they reach an internal temperature of 145°F (63°C).

For Sweet Potato Mash:

1. Boil or steam the diced sweet potatoes until they are fork-tender.
2. Drain the sweet potatoes and transfer them to a bowl.

3. Add unsalted butter, milk, salt, and pepper to the sweet potatoes.

4. Mash the sweet potatoes until smooth and creamy. Adjust the consistency with more milk if needed.

For Green Beans:

1. In a pan, heat olive oil over medium-high heat.

2. Add minced garlic to the pan and sauté for 1-2 minutes until fragrant.

3. Add trimmed green beans to the pan. Sauté for 5-7 minutes until the green beans are tender-crisp.

4. Season the green beans with salt and pepper to taste.

5. Optionally, sprinkle lemon zest over the green beans for added freshness.

To Serve:

1. Plate the grilled lean pork chops on each serving dish.

2. Serve with a side of sweet potato mash and sautéed green beans.

3. Optionally, garnish with additional dried thyme or a squeeze of lemon juice.

4. Enjoy this balanced and satisfying meal of grilled lean pork chops with sweet potato mash and green beans!

Baked chicken with lemon and rosemary, served with wild rice and roasted vegetables

Ingredients:

For Baked Chicken with Lemon and Rosemary:

- 4 bone-in, skin-on chicken thighs
- 2 tablespoons olive oil
- 2 tablespoons lemon juice
- 2 teaspoons fresh rosemary, chopped
- 2 cloves garlic, minced
- 1 teaspoon lemon zest
- Salt and pepper to taste
- Lemon slices for garnish

For Wild Rice:

- 1 cup wild rice
- 3 cups water or chicken broth
- 1/2 teaspoon salt

For Roasted Vegetables:

- 2 cups mixed vegetables (carrots, Brussels sprouts, cherry tomatoes, etc.), chopped
- 2 tablespoons olive oil
- 1 teaspoon dried thyme
- Salt and pepper to taste

Instructions:

For Baked Chicken with Lemon and Rosemary:

1. Preheat the oven to 400°F (200°C).
2. In a bowl, whisk together olive oil, lemon juice, chopped fresh rosemary, minced garlic, lemon zest, salt, and pepper.
3. Place the chicken thighs in a baking dish. Pour the lemon and rosemary mixture over the chicken, ensuring each thigh is well-coated.
4. Optionally, place lemon slices on top of each chicken thigh.
5. Bake in the preheated oven for 35-40 minutes or until the chicken reaches an internal temperature of 165°F (74°C) and the skin is crispy and golden.
6. Optionally, garnish with additional fresh rosemary and lemon slices before serving.

For Wild Rice:

1. In a saucepan, combine wild rice, water or chicken broth, and salt.
2. Bring to a boil, then reduce the heat to low, cover, and simmer for about 45-50 minutes or until the wild rice is tender and the liquid is absorbed.
3. Fluff the wild rice with a fork.

For Roasted Vegetables:

1. Preheat the oven to 400°F (200°C).
2. In a bowl, toss chopped mixed vegetables with olive oil, dried thyme, salt, and pepper until evenly coated.
3. Spread the vegetables on a baking sheet in a single layer.
4. Roast in the preheated oven for 20-25 minutes or until the vegetables are golden brown and tender, stirring halfway through.

To Serve:

1. Plate the baked chicken thighs on each serving dish.
2. Serve with a side of wild rice and roasted vegetables.
3. Optionally, garnish with additional fresh rosemary and lemon slices.

4. Enjoy this flavorful and balanced meal of baked chicken with lemon and rosemary, served with wild rice and roasted vegetables!

Grilled salmon with quinoa salad (tomatoes, cucumber, and fresh herbs)

Ingredients:

For Grilled Salmon:

- 4 salmon filets
- 2 tablespoons olive oil
- 2 tablespoons lemon juice
- 2 cloves garlic, minced
- 1 teaspoon dried dill
- Salt and pepper to taste
- Lemon wedges for serving

For Quinoa Salad:

- 1 cup quinoa, rinsed
- 2 cups water or vegetable broth
- 1 cucumber, diced
- 1 cup cherry tomatoes, halved
- 1/4 cup fresh parsley, chopped
- 1/4 cup fresh mint, chopped
- 1/4 cup red onion, finely chopped

- 3 tablespoons extra-virgin olive oil
- 2 tablespoons lemon juice
- Salt and pepper to taste

Instructions:

For Grilled Salmon:

1. Preheat the grill to medium-high heat.

2. In a bowl, whisk together olive oil, lemon juice, minced garlic, dried dill, salt, and pepper.

3. Place the salmon filets in a shallow dish. Pour the marinade over the salmon, ensuring each filet is well-coated. Let it marinate for at least 15-20 minutes.

4. Grill the salmon filets for 4-5 minutes per side or until they reach an internal temperature of 145°F (63°C) and the fish flakes easily with a fork.

5. Optionally, serve with lemon wedges.

For Quinoa Salad:

1. In a saucepan, combine rinsed quinoa, water or vegetable broth, and a pinch of salt.

2. Bring to a boil, then reduce the heat to low, cover, and simmer for about 15 minutes or until the quinoa is cooked and the liquid is absorbed.

3. Fluff the quinoa with a fork and let it cool to room temperature.

4. In a large bowl, combine cooked quinoa, diced cucumber, halved cherry tomatoes, chopped fresh parsley, chopped fresh mint, and finely chopped red onion.

5. In a small bowl, whisk together extra-virgin olive oil, lemon juice, salt, and pepper.

6. Pour the dressing over the quinoa salad and toss until all ingredients are well combined.

To Serve:

1. Plate the grilled salmon filets on each serving dish.

2. Serve with a generous portion of quinoa salad on the side.

3. Optionally, garnish with additional fresh herbs.

4. Enjoy this light and nutritious meal of grilled salmon with quinoa salad, featuring the freshness of tomatoes, cucumber, and herbs!

Baked cod with a citrus glaze, served with sweet potato wedges and steamed broccoli

Ingredients:
For Baked Cod with Citrus Glaze:

- 4 cod filets
- 2 tablespoons olive oil
- 2 tablespoons orange juice
- 1 tablespoon lemon juice
- 2 cloves garlic, minced
- 1 tablespoon honey
- 1 teaspoon Dijon mustard
- Salt and pepper to taste
- Fresh parsley for garnish

For Sweet Potato Wedges:

- 2 large sweet potatoes, peeled and cut into wedges
- 2 tablespoons olive oil
- 1 teaspoon smoked paprika
- 1 teaspoon cumin
- Salt and pepper to taste

For Steamed Broccoli:

- 2 cups broccoli florets
- 1 tablespoon olive oil
- Lemon zest (optional)
- Salt and pepper to taste

Instructions:

For Baked Cod with Citrus Glaze:

1. Preheat the oven to 400°F (200°C).

2. In a bowl, whisk together olive oil, orange juice, lemon juice, minced garlic, honey, Dijon mustard, salt, and pepper.

3. Place the cod filets in a baking dish. Pour the citrus glaze over the cod, ensuring each filet is well-coated.

4. Bake in the preheated oven for 15-20 minutes or until the cod is opaque and flakes easily with a fork.

5. Optionally, garnish with fresh parsley.

For Sweet Potato Wedges:

1. In a bowl, toss sweet potato wedges with olive oil, smoked paprika, cumin, salt, and pepper until evenly coated.

2. Spread the sweet potato wedges on a baking sheet in a single layer.

3. Roast in the preheated oven for 25-30 minutes or until the sweet potato wedges are tender and lightly browned, stirring halfway through.

For Steamed Broccoli:

1. In a steamer basket or a microwave-safe dish, place broccoli florets.

2. Steam in the steamer basket or microwave for 3-5 minutes or until the broccoli is tender but still crisp.
3. Drizzle olive oil over the steamed broccoli and season with salt and pepper to taste.
4. Optionally, sprinkle lemon zest over the broccoli for added freshness.

To Serve:
1. Plate the baked cod filets on each serving dish.
2. Serve with a side of sweet potato wedges and steamed broccoli.
3. Optionally, garnish with additional fresh parsley.
4. Enjoy this flavorful and balanced meal of baked cod with a citrus glaze, served with sweet potato wedges and steamed broccoli!

Grilled chicken breast with a side of wild rice and roasted Brussels sprouts

Ingredients:

For Grilled Chicken Breast:
- 4 boneless, skinless chicken breasts
- 2 tablespoons olive oil
- 2 teaspoons dried thyme
- 1 teaspoon paprika

- 1 teaspoon garlic powder
- Salt and pepper to taste
- Lemon wedges for serving

For Wild Rice:

- 1 cup wild rice
- 3 cups water or chicken broth
- 1/2 teaspoon salt

For Roasted Brussels Sprouts:

- 1 pound Brussels sprouts, trimmed and halved
- 2 tablespoons olive oil
- 1 teaspoon garlic powder
- Salt and pepper to taste

Instructions:

For Grilled Chicken Breast:

1. Preheat the grill to medium-high heat.
2. In a bowl, mix together olive oil, dried thyme, paprika, garlic powder, salt, and pepper.
3. Pat the chicken breasts dry with a paper towel. Brush the chicken breasts with the thyme and paprika mixture, ensuring each breast is well-coated.
4. Grill the chicken breasts for 6-7 minutes per side or until they reach an internal temperature of 165°F (74°C) and the juices run clear.

5. Optionally, serve with lemon wedges.

For Wild Rice:

1. In a saucepan, combine wild rice, water or chicken broth, and salt.

2. Bring to a boil, then reduce the heat to low, cover, and simmer for about 45-50 minutes or until the wild rice is tender and the liquid is absorbed.

3. Fluff the wild rice with a fork.

For Roasted Brussels Sprouts:

1. Preheat the oven to 400°F (200°C).

2. In a bowl, toss halved Brussels sprouts with olive oil, garlic powder, salt, and pepper until evenly coated.

3. Spread the Brussels sprouts on a baking sheet in a single layer.

4. Roast in the preheated oven for 20-25 minutes or until the Brussels sprouts are golden brown and crispy on the edges.

To Serve:

1. Plate the grilled chicken breasts on each serving dish.

2. Serve with a side of wild rice and roasted Brussels sprouts.

3. Optionally, garnish with additional dried thyme or a squeeze of lemon juice.

4. Enjoy this wholesome and balanced meal of grilled chicken breast with wild rice and roasted Brussels sprouts!

Baked turkey cutlets with a cranberry-orange glaze, quinoa, and roasted sweet potatoes

Ingredients:

For Baked Turkey Cutlets:

- 4 turkey cutlets
- 2 tablespoons olive oil
- 1 teaspoon dried thyme
- 1 teaspoon smoked paprika
- Salt and pepper to taste

For Cranberry-Orange Glaze:

- 1 cup cranberry sauce (homemade or store-bought)
- 1/4 cup orange juice
- 2 tablespoons honey
- 1 teaspoon grated orange zest

For Quinoa:

- 1 cup quinoa, rinsed
- 2 cups water or vegetable broth
- 1/2 teaspoon salt

For Roasted Sweet Potatoes:

- 2 large sweet potatoes, peeled and diced
- 2 tablespoons olive oil
- 1 teaspoon cinnamon
- 1/2 teaspoon nutmeg
- Salt to taste

Instructions:

For Baked Turkey Cutlets:

1. Preheat the oven to 400°F (200°C).
2. In a bowl, mix together olive oil, dried thyme, smoked paprika, salt, and pepper.
3. Place the turkey cutlets on a baking sheet lined with parchment paper or a greased baking dish. Brush the turkey cutlets with the spice mixture, ensuring each cutlet is well-coated.
4. Bake in the preheated oven for 20-25 minutes or until the turkey cutlets are cooked through.

For Cranberry-Orange Glaze:

1. In a saucepan, combine cranberry sauce, orange juice, honey, and grated orange zest.

2. Heat over medium heat, stirring frequently, until the mixture is well combined and heated through. Set aside.

For Quinoa:

1. In a saucepan, combine quinoa, water or vegetable broth, and salt.

2. Bring to a boil, then reduce the heat to low, cover, and simmer for about 15 minutes or until the quinoa is cooked and the liquid is absorbed.

3. Fluff the quinoa with a fork.

For Roasted Sweet Potatoes:

1. Preheat the oven to 400°F (200°C).

2. In a bowl, toss diced sweet potatoes with olive oil, cinnamon, nutmeg, and salt until evenly coated.

3. Spread the sweet potatoes on a baking sheet in a single layer.

4. Roast in the preheated oven for 25-30 minutes or until the sweet potatoes are tender and lightly browned, stirring halfway through.

To Serve:

1. Plate the baked turkey cutlets on each serving dish.

2. Drizzle the cranberry-orange glaze over the turkey cutlets.

3. Serve with a side of quinoa and roasted sweet potatoes.

4. Optionally, garnish with additional fresh thyme or orange zest.

5. Enjoy this festive and flavorful meal of baked turkey cutlets with a cranberry-orange glaze, quinoa, and roasted sweet potatoes!

Stir-fried tofu with bok choy and brown rice

Ingredients:

For Stir-Fried Tofu:
- 14 oz (400g) firm tofu, pressed and cubed
- 2 tablespoons soy sauce (low-sodium)
- 1 tablespoon hoisin sauce
- 1 tablespoon rice vinegar
- 1 tablespoon sesame oil
- 1 tablespoon cornstarch
- 2 tablespoons vegetable oil for stir-frying
- 2 cloves garlic, minced
- 1 tablespoon fresh ginger, grated
- Red pepper flakes (optional for heat)

For Bok Choy:

- 4 baby bok choy, chopped
- 2 tablespoons vegetable oil
- 2 cloves garlic, minced
- 1 tablespoon soy sauce (low-sodium)
- 1 tablespoon water

For Brown Rice:

- 1 cup brown rice
- 2 cups water
- 1/2 teaspoon salt

Instructions:

For Stir-Fried Tofu:

1. In a bowl, mix soy sauce, hoisin sauce, rice vinegar, sesame oil, and cornstarch to create the marinade.
2. Add the cubed tofu to the marinade, ensuring each piece is well-coated. Let it marinate for at least 15-20 minutes.
3. Heat vegetable oil in a wok or large skillet over medium-high heat.
4. Add minced garlic and grated ginger to the hot oil. Sauté for about 1-2 minutes until fragrant.

5. Add marinated tofu to the wok. Stir-fry for 5-7 minutes or until the tofu is golden brown and crispy.

6. Optionally, sprinkle red pepper flakes for added heat.

For Bok Choy:

1. In a separate pan, heat vegetable oil over medium heat.

2. Add minced garlic to the pan. Sauté for 1-2 minutes until fragrant.

3. Add chopped bok choy to the pan. Stir-fry for 3-5 minutes until the bok choy is wilted but still crisp.

4. Pour soy sauce and water over the bok choy. Toss to combine.

For Brown Rice:

1. In a saucepan, combine brown rice, water, and salt.

2. Bring to a boil, then reduce the heat to low, cover, and simmer for about 45-50 minutes or until the brown rice is tender and the liquid is absorbed.

3. Fluff the brown rice with a fork.

To Serve:

1. Plate the stir-fried tofu on each serving dish.

2. Serve with a side of bok choy and brown rice.

3. Optionally, garnish with chopped green onions or sesame seeds.

4. Enjoy this wholesome and plant-based stir-fried tofu with bok choy and brown rice!

Grilled shrimp with a side of wild rice and roasted Brussels sprouts

Ingredients:

For Grilled Shrimp:

- 1 pound large shrimp, peeled and deveined
- 2 tablespoons olive oil
- 2 cloves garlic, minced
- 1 teaspoon paprika
- 1 teaspoon dried oregano
- Salt and pepper to taste
- Lemon wedges for serving

For Wild Rice:

- 1 cup wild rice
- 3 cups water or vegetable broth
- 1/2 teaspoon salt

For Roasted Brussels Sprouts:

- 1 pound Brussels sprouts, trimmed and halved
- 2 tablespoons olive oil
- 1 teaspoon garlic powder
- Salt and pepper to taste

Instructions:

For Grilled Shrimp:

1. Preheat the grill to medium-high heat.
2. In a bowl, mix together olive oil, minced garlic, paprika, dried oregano, salt, and pepper.
3. Toss the peeled and deveined shrimp in the marinade until well-coated.
4. Thread the shrimp onto skewers.
5. Grill the shrimp skewers for 2-3 minutes per side or until they are opaque and cooked through.
6. Optionally, serve with lemon wedges.

For Wild Rice:

1. In a saucepan, combine wild rice, water or vegetable broth, and salt.
2. Bring to a boil, then reduce the heat to low, cover, and simmer for about 45-50 minutes or until the wild rice is tender and the liquid is absorbed.

3. Fluff the wild rice with a fork.

For Roasted Brussels Sprouts:

1. Preheat the oven to 400°F (200°C).

2. In a bowl, toss halved Brussels sprouts with olive oil, garlic powder, salt, and pepper until evenly coated.

3. Spread the Brussels sprouts on a baking sheet in a single layer.

4. Roast in the preheated oven for 20-25 minutes or until the Brussels sprouts are golden brown and crispy on the edges, stirring halfway through.

To Serve:

1. Plate the grilled shrimp skewers on each serving dish.

2. Serve with a side of wild rice and roasted Brussels sprouts.

3. Optionally, garnish with fresh chopped parsley or a squeeze of lemon juice.

4. Enjoy this delicious and balanced meal of grilled shrimp with wild rice and roasted Brussels sprouts!

"I trust my body's wisdom to digest and absorb nutrients effectively, promoting optimal health."

"I am empowered to make choices that contribute to my well-being, both physically and mentally."

CHAPTER 5: SNACKS AND APPETIZERS

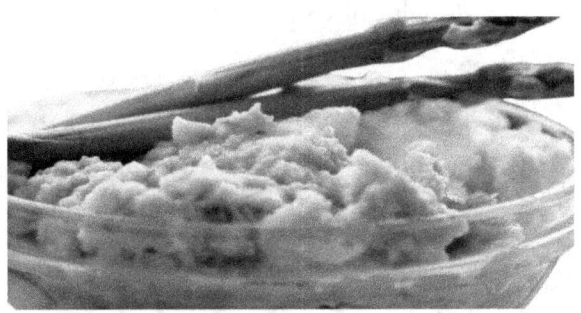

Asparagus Guacamole

Ingredients:

- 1 bunch fresh asparagus, trimmed
- 2 ripe avocados, peeled and pitted
- 1/2 cup cherry tomatoes, halved
- 1/4 cup red onion, finely diced
- 1 clove garlic, minced
- 1 lime, juiced
- 2 tablespoons fresh cilantro, chopped
- Salt and pepper to taste
- Optional: Jalapeño slices for heat
- Tortilla chips or vegetable sticks for serving

Instructions:

1. Preheat the oven to 400°F (200°C).

2. Place trimmed asparagus on a baking sheet. Drizzle with olive oil and season with salt and pepper.

3. Roast the asparagus in the preheated oven for 10-15 minutes or until tender but still slightly crisp. Let it cool.

4. In a medium bowl, mash the ripe avocados with a fork.

5. Cut the roasted asparagus into small pieces and add them to the mashed avocados.

6. Add halved cherry tomatoes, finely diced red onion, minced garlic, lime juice, and chopped cilantro to the bowl. Mix everything together.

7. Season the asparagus guacamole with salt and pepper to taste. If you like it spicy, add jalapeño slices.

8. Refrigerate the guacamole for at least 30 minutes to allow the flavors to meld.

9. Before serving, give the guacamole a final stir and adjust the seasoning if needed.

10. Serve the asparagus guacamole with tortilla chips or vegetable sticks.

11. Enjoy this unique twist on guacamole, adding the freshness and flavor of roasted asparagus to the classic avocado dip!

Sliced bell peppers with hummus

Ingredients:

- 3 bell peppers (assorted colors), sliced
- 1 cup hummus (store-bought or homemade)
- 2 tablespoons olive oil
- 1 teaspoon lemon juice
- 1 clove garlic, minced
- Salt and pepper to taste
- Fresh parsley for garnish (optional)
- Pita bread or vegetable sticks for serving

Instructions:

1. Wash and slice the bell peppers into strips.
2. In a small bowl, whisk together olive oil, lemon juice, minced garlic, salt, and pepper to create a simple dressing.
3. Arrange the sliced bell peppers on a serving platter.
4. Drizzle the dressing over the sliced bell peppers.
5. In the center of the platter, place a bowl of hummus.

6. Optionally, garnish the hummus with a drizzle of olive oil and a sprinkle of fresh parsley.

7. Serve the sliced bell peppers with hummus alongside pita bread or vegetable sticks.

8. Enjoy this colorful and nutritious snack or appetizer with the delightful combination of sliced bell peppers and creamy hummus!

Paleo Sweet Potato Snack Bowl

Ingredients:

- 2 medium sweet potatoes, peeled and cubed
- 2 tablespoons coconut oil, melted
- 1 teaspoon cinnamon
- 1/2 teaspoon nutmeg
- Pinch of salt
- 1/4 cup unsweetened coconut flakes
- 1/4 cup chopped nuts (e.g., almonds, walnuts, pecans)
- 1/4 cup fresh berries (e.g., blueberries, raspberries, strawberries)
- 1 tablespoon chia seeds
- 1 tablespoon honey (optional)

Instructions:

1. Preheat the oven to 400°F (200°C).

2. In a large bowl, toss the cubed sweet potatoes with melted coconut oil, cinnamon, nutmeg, and a pinch of salt until evenly coated.

3. Spread the sweet potatoes on a baking sheet in a single layer.

4. Roast in the preheated oven for 20-25 minutes or until the sweet potatoes are tender and golden brown, stirring halfway through.

5. While the sweet potatoes are roasting, toast the coconut flakes and chopped nuts in a dry skillet over medium heat until they are lightly browned and fragrant. Keep an eye on them to prevent burning.

6. Once the sweet potatoes are done, transfer them to a serving bowl.

7. Top the roasted sweet potatoes with toasted coconut flakes, chopped nuts, fresh berries, and chia seeds.

8. Optionally, drizzle honey over the top for added sweetness.

9. Toss the ingredients together gently to combine.

10. Serve the Paleo Sweet Potato Snack Bowl immediately and enjoy this wholesome and satisfying snack that combines the natural sweetness of sweet potatoes with the crunch of coconut, nuts, and the freshness of berries!

Watermelon Fruit Bowl

Ingredients:

- 1 medium-sized watermelon
- 2 cups fresh strawberries, hulled and halved
- 1 cup fresh blueberries
- 1 cup fresh kiwi, peeled and diced
- 1 cup fresh pineapple, peeled and diced
- 1 cup fresh mango, peeled and diced
- 1 cup seedless grapes, halved
- 1 tablespoon fresh mint leaves, chopped
- 1 tablespoon honey (optional)
- Juice of 1 lime

Instructions:

1. Cut the watermelon in half lengthwise. Use a melon baller or a spoon to scoop out bite-sized watermelon balls from each half. Reserve the watermelon shells to use as bowls.

2. In a large mixing bowl, combine the watermelon balls, strawberries, blueberries, diced kiwi, diced pineapple, diced mango, and halved grapes.

3. Squeeze the juice of one lime over the fruit mixture. Optionally, drizzle honey over the fruit for added sweetness.

4. Toss the fruits gently to combine.

5. Arrange the fruit mixture inside the watermelon shells.

6. Sprinkle chopped mint leaves over the top for a burst of freshness.

7. Chill the Watermelon Fruit Bowl in the refrigerator for at least 30 minutes before serving.

8. Serve this refreshing and vibrant fruit bowl at your next gathering or enjoy it as a healthy and delightful snack.

9. Enjoy the juicy and colorful combination of watermelon, berries, and tropical fruits in this delicious Watermelon Fruit Bowl!

A handful of mixed berries with a dollop of low-fat yogurt

Ingredients:
- 1 cup mixed berries (e.g., strawberries, blueberries, raspberries, blackberries)
- 1/2 cup low-fat yogurt
- 1 tablespoon honey (optional)
- Fresh mint leaves for garnish (optional)

174

Instructions:

1. Wash the mixed berries thoroughly and pat them dry with a paper towel.
2. In a bowl or serving dish, arrange the mixed berries.
3. In the center of the berries, place a generous dollop of low-fat yogurt.
4. Optionally, drizzle honey over the berries and yogurt for added sweetness.
5. Garnish with fresh mint leaves for a burst of freshness.
6. Serve the Handful of Mixed Berries with a Dollop of Low-Fat Yogurt immediately.
7. Enjoy this simple and nutritious snack that combines the natural sweetness of berries with the creamy texture of low-fat yogurt!

Edamame with a sprinkle of sea salt

Ingredients:

- 2 cups edamame (fresh or frozen)
- 1 tablespoon sea salt (or to taste)

Instructions:

1. If using frozen edamame, thaw them according to the package instructions.

2. In a medium-sized pot, bring water to a boil. Add a pinch of salt to the boiling water.

3. Add the edamame to the boiling water and cook for about 5 minutes or until they are tender.

4. Drain the edamame and transfer them to a serving bowl.

5. While the edamame are still hot, sprinkle sea salt over them. Toss the edamame to ensure even coating with salt.

6. Serve the Edamame with a Sprinkle of Sea Salt immediately.

7. Enjoy this simple and protein-packed snack that highlights the natural flavor of edamame with a touch of sea salt!

Roasted Sweet Potato

Ingredients:

- 3 medium-sized sweet potatoes, peeled and cubed
- 2 tablespoons olive oil
- 1 teaspoon smoked paprika
- 1 teaspoon garlic powder
- 1 teaspoon ground cumin
- Salt and pepper to taste

- Fresh parsley for garnish (optional)

Instructions:

1. Preheat the oven to 400°F (200°C).

2. In a large bowl, toss the cubed sweet potatoes with olive oil, smoked paprika, garlic powder, ground cumin, salt, and pepper until evenly coated.

3. Spread the seasoned sweet potatoes on a baking sheet in a single layer.

4. Roast in the preheated oven for 25-30 minutes or until the sweet potatoes are tender and caramelized, stirring halfway through.

5. Once the sweet potatoes are done, transfer them to a serving dish.

6. Optionally, garnish with fresh chopped parsley for a burst of freshness.

7. Serve the Roasted Sweet Potatoes immediately.

8. Enjoy this simple and flavorful side dish that brings out the natural sweetness of sweet potatoes with a hint of smokiness and spice!

Carrot and cucumber sticks with tzatziki

Ingredients:

For Tzatziki:

- 1 cup Greek yogurt
- 1/2 cucumber, finely grated and drained
- 2 cloves garlic, minced
- 1 tablespoon fresh dill, chopped
- 1 tablespoon fresh mint, chopped
- 1 tablespoon extra-virgin olive oil
- 1 tablespoon lemon juice
- Salt and pepper to taste

For Carrot and Cucumber Sticks:

- 3 large carrots, peeled and cut into sticks
- 2 cucumbers, cut into sticks

Instructions:

For Tzatziki:

1. In a bowl, combine Greek yogurt, grated and drained cucumber, minced garlic, chopped fresh dill, chopped fresh mint, olive oil, lemon juice, salt, and pepper.
2. Mix all the ingredients until well combined.
3. Refrigerate the tzatziki for at least 30 minutes to allow the flavors to meld.

For Carrot and Cucumber Sticks:

1. Wash, peel, and cut the carrots into sticks.

2. Wash and cut the cucumbers into sticks.

3. Arrange the carrot and cucumber sticks on a serving platter.

4. Serve the tzatziki alongside the carrot and cucumber sticks.

5. Optionally, garnish the tzatziki with a drizzle of olive oil and a sprinkle of fresh herbs.

6. Enjoy this refreshing and crunchy snack of carrot and cucumber sticks with creamy tzatziki dip!

Chia seed pudding with berries

Ingredients:

- 1/4 cup chia seeds
- 1 cup almond milk (or any milk of your choice)
- 1 tablespoon maple syrup or honey
- 1/2 teaspoon vanilla extract
- Mixed berries (e.g., strawberries, blueberries, raspberries) for topping
- Optional toppings: sliced almonds, shredded coconut, mint leaves

Instructions:

1. In a bowl, combine chia seeds, almond milk, maple syrup (or honey), and vanilla extract.

2. Whisk the mixture well to ensure the chia seeds are evenly distributed. Let it sit for a few minutes.

3. After about 5 minutes, whisk the mixture again to prevent clumping, making sure the chia seeds are well incorporated.

4. Cover the bowl and refrigerate the chia seed mixture for at least 3 hours or overnight to allow it to thicken.

5. Once the chia pudding has set, give it a good stir to break up any clumps.

6. Spoon the chia pudding into serving glasses or bowls.

7. Top the chia pudding with mixed berries.

8. Optionally, garnish with additional toppings like sliced almonds, shredded coconut, or mint leaves.

9. Serve the Chia Seed Pudding with Berries immediately or refrigerate until ready to enjoy.

10. This chia seed pudding is a delicious and nutritious breakfast or snack, combining the creamy texture of chia seeds with the sweetness of berries!

Dry-Roasted Chickpea

Ingredients:

- 1 can (15 oz) chickpeas (garbanzo beans), drained and rinsed
- 1 tablespoon olive oil
- 1 teaspoon ground cumin
- 1 teaspoon smoked paprika
- 1/2 teaspoon garlic powder
- 1/2 teaspoon chili powder
- 1/2 teaspoon cayenne pepper (adjust to taste)
- Salt to taste

Instructions:

1. Preheat the oven to 400°F (200°C).

2. Rinse and drain the chickpeas. Pat them dry with a paper towel to remove excess moisture.

3. In a bowl, toss the chickpeas with olive oil, ground cumin, smoked paprika, garlic powder, chili powder, cayenne pepper, and salt until well coated.

4. Spread the seasoned chickpeas in a single layer on a baking sheet lined with parchment paper.

5. Roast in the preheated oven for 25-30 minutes or until the chickpeas are golden brown and crispy, shaking the pan halfway through for even roasting.

6. Remove the chickpeas from the oven and let them cool slightly.

7. Serve the Dry-Roasted Chickpeas as a crunchy snack or a protein-packed topping for salads.

8. Enjoy this simple and flavorful snack that brings out the nutty taste and crispiness of roasted chickpeas!

Ginger Tahini Dip With Assorted Veggies

Ingredients:

For Ginger Tahini Dip:
- 1/2 cup tahini
- 2 tablespoons fresh lemon juice
- 1 tablespoon tamari or soy sauce
- 1 tablespoon pure maple syrup
- 1 teaspoon grated fresh ginger
- 1 clove garlic, minced
- 2 tablespoons water (adjust for desired consistency)
- Salt and pepper to taste

For Assorted Veggies:
- Carrot sticks
- Cucumber slices

- Bell pepper strips (assorted colors)
- Cherry tomatoes, halved
- Radishes, sliced

Instructions:

For Ginger Tahini Dip:

1. In a bowl, whisk together tahini, fresh lemon juice, tamari or soy sauce, pure maple syrup, grated fresh ginger, minced garlic, water, salt, and pepper.
2. Adjust the consistency by adding more water if needed. The dip should be smooth and creamy.
3. Taste and adjust the seasoning according to your preference.
4. Refrigerate the Ginger Tahini Dip for at least 30 minutes to allow the flavors to meld.

For Assorted Veggies:

1. Wash, peel (if necessary), and cut the vegetables into sticks, slices, or strips.
2. Arrange the assorted veggies on a serving platter.
3. Take the Ginger Tahini Dip out of the refrigerator.
4. Serve the dip alongside the assorted veggies.

5. Enjoy this nutritious and flavorful snack that combines the creamy richness of tahini with the freshness of assorted veggies!

Mixed nuts and dried fruit trail mix

Ingredients:
- 1 cup almonds
- 1 cup walnuts
- 1 cup cashews
- 1 cup pistachios (shelled)
- 1 cup dried cranberries
- 1 cup dried apricots, chopped
- 1/2 cup raisins
- 1/2 cup dried blueberries
- 1/2 cup dark chocolate chips (optional)
- 1 teaspoon ground cinnamon (optional)

Instructions:
1. Preheat the oven to 350°F (175°C).
2. In a large mixing bowl, combine almonds, walnuts, cashews, and pistachios.
3. Spread the mixed nuts on a baking sheet in a single layer.

4. Roast the nuts in the preheated oven for 10-12 minutes or until they are fragrant and lightly toasted. Stir occasionally for even roasting.

5. Remove the nuts from the oven and let them cool completely.

6. Once the nuts are cooled, add dried cranberries, chopped dried apricots, raisins, dried blueberries, and dark chocolate chips to the mixing bowl.

7. Optionally, sprinkle ground cinnamon over the mixture for added flavor.

8. Toss all the ingredients together until they are well combined.

9. Store the Mixed Nuts and Dried Fruit Trail Mix in an airtight container.

10. Enjoy this homemade trail mix as a convenient and energy-boosting snack on the go or a satisfying topping for yogurt or oatmeal!

Sliced apple with almond butter

Ingredients:

- 2 medium-sized apples (e.g., Honeycrisp, Gala), cored and sliced
- 1/2 cup almond butter

- 1 tablespoon honey (optional)
- 1/2 teaspoon ground cinnamon (optional)
- Sliced almonds for garnish (optional)

Instructions:

1. Wash, core, and slice the apples into thin rounds or wedges.

2. In a small microwave-safe bowl, gently heat the almond butter for 15-20 seconds until it becomes slightly more spreadable.

3. Arrange the apple slices on a serving plate.

4. Drizzle almond butter over the apple slices using a spoon or transfer the almond butter to a small bowl for dipping.

5. Optionally, drizzle honey over the almond butter for added sweetness.

6. If desired, sprinkle ground cinnamon over the almond butter.

7. Optionally, garnish with sliced almonds for extra crunch.

8. Serve the Sliced Apple with Almond Butter immediately.

9. Enjoy this simple and nutritious snack that combines the crispness of apples with the creamy richness of almond butter!

Taro Chips

Ingredients:

- 2 large taro roots, peeled and thinly sliced
- 2 tablespoons olive oil
- Salt to taste
- Optional: Paprika, garlic powder, or other desired seasonings

Instructions:

1. Preheat the oven to 375°F (190°C).
2. Peel the taro roots and thinly slice them using a mandoline or a sharp knife.
3. In a large bowl, toss the taro slices with olive oil until they are evenly coated.
4. Arrange the taro slices in a single layer on baking sheets lined with parchment paper.
5. Sprinkle salt over the taro slices. Optionally, add paprika, garlic powder, or other desired seasonings for additional flavor.
6. Bake in the preheated oven for 20-25 minutes or until the taro chips are golden brown and crisp. Flip the chips halfway through the baking time for even cooking.
7. Once the taro chips are done, remove them from the oven and let them cool on the baking sheets.

8. Store the Taro Chips in an airtight container once they are completely cooled.

9. Enjoy this crunchy and flavorful snack as a healthier alternative to traditional potato chips!

Carrot sticks with hummus

Ingredients:

- 4 large carrots, peeled and cut into sticks
- 1 cup hummus (store-bought or homemade)
- 2 tablespoons olive oil
- 1 teaspoon ground cumin
- 1/2 teaspoon smoked paprika
- Salt and pepper to taste
- Fresh parsley for garnish (optional)

Instructions:

1. Wash, peel, and cut the carrots into sticks.
2. In a small bowl, mix olive oil, ground cumin, smoked paprika, salt, and pepper.
3. Toss the carrot sticks in the spice mixture until they are well coated.
4. Arrange the spiced carrot sticks on a serving platter.
5. In the center of the platter, place a bowl of hummus.

6. Optionally, drizzle olive oil over the hummus and sprinkle fresh parsley for garnish.
7. Serve the Carrot Sticks with Hummus immediately.
8. Enjoy this simple and nutritious snack that combines the sweetness of carrots with the creamy richness of hummus!

Sweet Potato Chips

Ingredients:

- 2 medium-sized sweet potatoes, peeled
- 2 tablespoons olive oil
- 1 teaspoon smoked paprika
- 1/2 teaspoon garlic powder
- 1/2 teaspoon sea salt
- Freshly ground black pepper to taste

Instructions:

1. Preheat the oven to 375°F (190°C).
2. Using a mandoline slicer or a sharp knife, thinly slice the peeled sweet potatoes into uniform rounds.
3. In a large bowl, toss the sweet potato slices with olive oil, smoked paprika, garlic powder, sea salt, and freshly ground black pepper until the slices are evenly coated.
4. Line baking sheets with parchment paper.

5. Arrange the seasoned sweet potato slices in a single layer on the prepared baking sheets, ensuring they are not overlapping.

6. Bake in the preheated oven for 15-20 minutes or until the sweet potato chips are golden brown and crispy. Keep an eye on them to prevent burning.

7. Once done, remove the sweet potato chips from the oven and let them cool on the baking sheets.

8. Allow the Sweet Potato Chips to cool completely before serving.

9. Store the cooled chips in an airtight container for later use.

10. Enjoy these homemade sweet potato chips as a healthier alternative to traditional potato chips!

Grain-Free Mixed Seed Crackers

Ingredients:

- 1 cup almond flour
- 2 tablespoons flaxseed meal
- 2 tablespoons chia seeds
- 2 tablespoons sesame seeds
- 2 tablespoons sunflower seeds
- 2 tablespoons pumpkin seeds

- 1/2 teaspoon salt
- 1/2 teaspoon garlic powder
- 1/2 teaspoon dried oregano
- 1/4 teaspoon black pepper
- 1/4 cup water
- 1 tablespoon olive oil

Instructions:

1. Preheat the oven to 325°F (163°C). Line a baking sheet with parchment paper.
2. In a large mixing bowl, combine almond flour, flaxseed meal, chia seeds, sesame seeds, sunflower seeds, pumpkin seeds, salt, garlic powder, dried oregano, and black pepper.
3. In a separate small bowl, mix water and olive oil.
4. Pour the wet ingredients into the dry ingredients and stir until a dough forms. Let the mixture sit for a couple of minutes to allow the chia seeds to absorb some of the liquid.
5. Place the dough on the prepared baking sheet and cover it with another piece of parchment paper.
6. Roll out the dough between the two sheets of parchment paper until it forms a thin, even layer.

7. Remove the top parchment paper, and use a knife or pizza cutter to score the dough into desired cracker shapes.

8. Bake in the preheated oven for 20-25 minutes or until the edges are golden brown and the crackers are firm to the touch.

9. Remove from the oven and let it cool on the baking sheet.

10. Once cooled, break the crackers along the scored lines.

11. Store the Grain-Free Mixed Seed Crackers in an airtight container.

12. Enjoy these homemade, nutrient-packed crackers as a grain-free and gluten-free snack!

Cottage cheese with pineapple chunks

Ingredients:
- 1 cup cottage cheese
- 1 cup fresh pineapple chunks (or canned pineapple chunks, drained)
- 1 tablespoon honey (optional)
- Mint leaves for garnish (optional)

Instructions:
1. In a serving bowl, place the cottage cheese.

2. Add the fresh pineapple chunks to the cottage cheese.
3. Optionally, drizzle honey over the cottage cheese and pineapple for added sweetness.
4. Gently toss the cottage cheese and pineapple together.
5. Garnish with mint leaves for a fresh touch (optional).
6. Serve the Cottage Cheese with Pineapple immediately.
7. Enjoy this simple and satisfying snack that combines the creamy texture of cottage cheese with the tropical sweetness of pineapple!

Greek yogurt with a handful of mixed nuts

Ingredients:
- 1 cup Greek yogurt
- 1/4 cup mixed nuts (e.g., almonds, walnuts, pistachios), chopped
- 1 tablespoon honey (optional)
- Fresh berries for garnish (optional)

Instructions:
1. Spoon the Greek yogurt into a serving bowl.

2. Sprinkle the mixed nuts over the Greek yogurt.

3. Optionally, drizzle honey over the yogurt and nuts for added sweetness.

4. Garnish with fresh berries for a burst of color and flavor (optional).

5. Serve the Greek Yogurt with a Handful of Mixed Nuts immediately.

6. Enjoy this protein-packed and satisfying snack that combines the creaminess of Greek yogurt with the crunch of mixed nuts!

Cajun Baked French Fries

Ingredients:

- 4 medium-sized russet potatoes, washed and cut into fries
- 2 tablespoons olive oil
- 1 tablespoon Cajun seasoning
- 1/2 teaspoon garlic powder
- 1/2 teaspoon onion powder
- 1/2 teaspoon paprika
- 1/2 teaspoon dried thyme
- 1/2 teaspoon dried oregano
- Salt and pepper to taste
- Fresh parsley for garnish (optional)

Instructions:

1. Preheat the oven to 425°F (220°C). Line a baking sheet with parchment paper.

2. In a large bowl, combine olive oil, Cajun seasoning, garlic powder, onion powder, paprika, dried thyme, dried oregano, salt, and pepper.

3. Add the cut potatoes to the bowl and toss them until they are evenly coated with the Cajun seasoning mixture.

4. Spread the seasoned potato fries in a single layer on the prepared baking sheet.

5. Bake in the preheated oven for 25-30 minutes or until the fries are golden brown and crispy, flipping them halfway through for even cooking.

6. Once the Cajun Baked French Fries are done, remove them from the oven and let them cool slightly.

7. Optionally, garnish with fresh chopped parsley for added freshness.

8. Serve the Cajun Baked French Fries immediately.

9. Enjoy this flavorful twist on traditional fries with the bold Cajun seasoning!

Sliced apple with a small portion of cheese

Ingredients:

- 2 medium-sized apples (e.g., Honeycrisp, Granny Smith), cored and sliced
- 1/2 cup cheese (e.g., sharp cheddar, Gouda, Brie), sliced or cubed
- 1 tablespoon honey or maple syrup (optional)
- 1/4 cup chopped nuts (e.g., walnuts, pecans) for garnish (optional)

Instructions:

1. Wash, core, and slice the apples into thin rounds or wedges.
2. Arrange the apple slices on a serving plate.
3. Place slices or cubes of your chosen cheese next to the apple slices.
4. Optionally, drizzle honey or maple syrup over the cheese and apples for added sweetness.
5. If desired, sprinkle chopped nuts over the top for added crunch.

6. Serve the Sliced Apple with a Small Portion of Cheese immediately.

7. Enjoy this simple and balanced snack that combines the natural sweetness of apples with the savory richness of cheese!

Mixed nuts and dried apricots

Ingredients:

- 1 cup mixed nuts (e.g., almonds, walnuts, cashews)
- 1/2 cup dried apricots, chopped

Instructions:

1. If the nuts are raw, you can toast them for added flavor. Place them in a dry skillet over medium heat and stir frequently until they become fragrant and lightly browned. Be careful not to burn them. Alternatively, you can use pre-roasted nuts.

2. Let the nuts cool completely before proceeding.

3. In a bowl, combine the mixed nuts and chopped dried apricots.

4. Toss the nuts and dried apricots together until they are well mixed.

5. Serve the Mixed Nuts and Dried Apricots immediately.

6. Enjoy this simple and nutritious snack that combines the crunch of mixed nuts with the natural sweetness of dried apricots!

Handful of walnuts and a small bunch of grapes

Ingredients:

- 1 handful of walnuts
- 1 small bunch of grapes (red or green)

Instructions:

1. Wash the grapes thoroughly and pat them dry with a paper towel.
2. Arrange the walnuts and grapes on a serving plate.
3. Serve the Handful of Walnuts and a Small Bunch of Grapes immediately.
4. Enjoy this quick and nutritious snack that combines the earthy flavor of walnuts with the sweet juiciness of grapes!

"Balanced meals bring balance to my body, mind, and spirit."

"I listen to my body and provide it with the care it deserves."

CHAPTER 6: MAIN COURSES

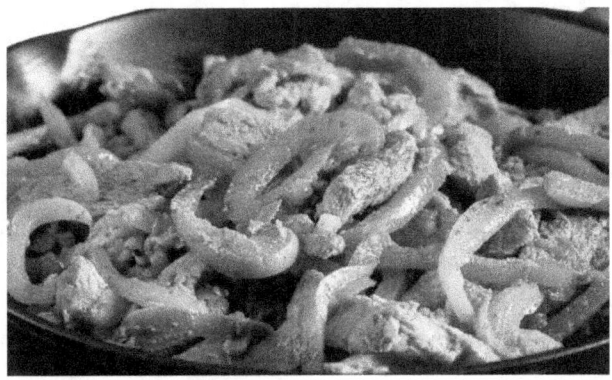

Couscous Salad

Ingredients:

- 1 cup couscous
- 1 1/4 cups vegetable or chicken broth
- 1 cup cherry tomatoes, halved
- 1 cucumber, diced
- 1/2 cup red bell pepper, diced
- 1/4 cup red onion, finely chopped
- 1/4 cup Kalamata olives, sliced
- 1/4 cup feta cheese, crumbled
- 3 tablespoons extra-virgin olive oil
- 2 tablespoons fresh lemon juice
- 1 teaspoon Dijon mustard
- 1 clove garlic, minced

- 1 teaspoon dried oregano
- Salt and black pepper to taste
- Fresh parsley for garnish (optional)

Instructions:

1. In a medium saucepan, bring the broth to a boil. Stir in the couscous, cover the pan, and remove it from heat. Let it sit for 5 minutes to allow the couscous to absorb the liquid.
2. Fluff the couscous with a fork to separate the grains. Allow it to cool to room temperature.
3. In a large bowl, combine the cooled couscous, cherry tomatoes, cucumber, red bell pepper, red onion, Kalamata olives, and feta cheese.
4. In a small bowl, whisk together the olive oil, lemon juice, Dijon mustard, minced garlic, dried oregano, salt, and black pepper to create the dressing.
5. Pour the dressing over the couscous mixture and toss until everything is well coated.
6. Taste and adjust the seasoning if necessary.
7. Optionally, garnish the Couscous Salad with fresh parsley.
8. Refrigerate for at least 30 minutes before serving to allow the flavors to meld.

9. Serve the Couscous Salad as a refreshing and flavorful side dish.

10. Enjoy this versatile and colorful salad that can be served on its own or as a complement to grilled meats or seafood!

Sautéed Turkey With Cabbage

Ingredients:

- 1 pound ground turkey
- 1 small head of cabbage, shredded
- 1 onion, finely chopped
- 2 cloves garlic, minced
- 1 teaspoon ground cumin
- 1 teaspoon smoked paprika
- 1/2 teaspoon dried thyme
- Salt and black pepper to taste
- 2 tablespoons olive oil
- Fresh parsley for garnish (optional)

Instructions:

1. In a large skillet, heat olive oil over medium heat.

2. Add chopped onion and minced garlic to the skillet. Sauté until the onion becomes translucent.

3. Add ground turkey to the skillet, breaking it apart with a spatula. Cook until the turkey is browned and cooked through.

4. Sprinkle ground cumin, smoked paprika, dried thyme, salt, and black pepper over the turkey. Stir to combine and let the spices toast for a minute.

5. Add shredded cabbage to the skillet. Mix well with the turkey and spices.

6. Cover the skillet and cook for 10-15 minutes, stirring occasionally, until the cabbage is tender but still has a bit of crunch.

7. Taste and adjust the seasoning if necessary.

8. Optionally, garnish the Sautéed Turkey with Cabbage with fresh parsley for a burst of freshness.

9. Serve the sautéed turkey and cabbage mixture as a flavorful and low-carb main dish.

10. Enjoy this quick and healthy recipe that combines lean turkey with the vibrant crunch of cabbage!

Baked Lemon Salmon With Zucchini

Ingredients:

- 4 salmon filets
- 2 medium-sized zucchinis, sliced
- 3 tablespoons olive oil
- 2 tablespoons fresh lemon juice
- 2 teaspoons Dijon mustard
- 2 cloves garlic, minced
- 1 teaspoon dried oregano
- Salt and black pepper to taste
- Lemon slices for garnish
- Fresh parsley for garnish (optional)

Instructions:

1. Preheat the oven to 400°F (200°C). Line a baking sheet with parchment paper.
2. In a small bowl, whisk together olive oil, fresh lemon juice, Dijon mustard, minced garlic, dried oregano, salt, and black pepper to create the marinade.
3. Place the salmon filets and sliced zucchinis in a large bowl. Pour half of the marinade over them and toss to coat evenly.
4. Arrange the marinated salmon filets and zucchini slices on the prepared baking sheet.

5. Drizzle the remaining marinade over the salmon and zucchini.

6. Bake in the preheated oven for 15-20 minutes or until the salmon is cooked through and flakes easily with a fork, and the zucchini is tender.

7. Optionally, garnish with lemon slices and fresh parsley.

8. Serve the Baked Lemon Salmon with Zucchini immediately.

9. Enjoy this light and flavorful dish that pairs the citrusy goodness of lemon with the richness of baked salmon and tender zucchini!

Cajun Catfish

Ingredients:

- 4 catfish filets
- 2 tablespoons Cajun seasoning
- 1 teaspoon paprika
- 1/2 teaspoon garlic powder
- 1/2 teaspoon onion powder
- 1/2 teaspoon dried thyme
- 1/2 teaspoon dried oregano
- 1/4 teaspoon cayenne pepper (adjust to taste)
- Salt and black pepper to taste

- 2 tablespoons olive oil
- Lemon wedges for serving
- Fresh parsley for garnish (optional)

Instructions:

1. Preheat the oven to 400°F (200°C). Line a baking sheet with parchment paper.

2. In a small bowl, mix Cajun seasoning, paprika, garlic powder, onion powder, dried thyme, dried oregano, cayenne pepper, salt, and black pepper.

3. Pat the catfish filets dry with a paper towel. Rub both sides of each filet with the Cajun seasoning mixture, ensuring they are well coated.

4. Heat olive oil in an oven-safe skillet over medium-high heat.

5. Place the catfish filets in the skillet and sear for 2-3 minutes on each side until they develop a golden crust.

6. Transfer the skillet to the preheated oven and bake for an additional 8-10 minutes or until the catfish is cooked through and flakes easily with a fork.

7. Optionally, garnish with fresh parsley.

8. Serve the Cajun Catfish with lemon wedges on the side.

9. Enjoy this spicy and flavorful catfish dish that brings a taste of Cajun cuisine to your table!

Kale and Cottage Pasta

Ingredients:

- 8 oz whole wheat pasta (or pasta of your choice)
- 1 bunch kale, stems removed and leaves chopped
- 1 cup cottage cheese
- 2 tablespoons olive oil
- 3 cloves garlic, minced
- 1/4 teaspoon red pepper flakes (optional)
- Salt and black pepper to taste
- Grated Parmesan cheese for garnish (optional)

Instructions:

1. Cook the pasta according to the package instructions. Drain and set aside.
2. In a large skillet, heat olive oil over medium heat. Add minced garlic and red pepper flakes (if using) and sauté for about 1 minute until the garlic becomes fragrant.
3. Add the chopped kale to the skillet. Sauté for 3-5 minutes until the kale is wilted but still vibrant green.

4. Stir in the cooked pasta and cottage cheese. Mix well until the cottage cheese coats the pasta and kale evenly.

5. Season with salt and black pepper to taste. Adjust the seasoning as needed.

6. Cook for an additional 2-3 minutes until everything is heated through.

7. Optionally, garnish with grated Parmesan cheese.

8. Serve the Kale and Cottage Pasta immediately.

9. Enjoy this wholesome and flavorful pasta dish that combines the nutritional benefits of kale with the creamy texture of cottage cheese!

Chicken Fajita Bowl

Ingredients:

- 1 pound boneless, skinless chicken breasts, sliced into strips
- 2 bell peppers (any color), sliced
- 1 large red onion, sliced
- 2 tablespoons olive oil
- 1 teaspoon chili powder
- 1 teaspoon cumin
- 1/2 teaspoon smoked paprika

- 1/2 teaspoon garlic powder
- Salt and black pepper to taste
- Cooked brown rice or cauliflower rice for serving
- Optional toppings: salsa, guacamole, sour cream, shredded cheese, lime wedges, chopped cilantro

Instructions:

1. In a large bowl, combine sliced chicken, bell peppers, and red onion.
2. In a small bowl, mix together olive oil, chili powder, cumin, smoked paprika, garlic powder, salt, and black pepper to create the fajita seasoning.
3. Pour the fajita seasoning over the chicken and vegetables. Toss to coat evenly.
4. Heat a large skillet over medium-high heat. Add the chicken and vegetable mixture to the skillet.
5. Cook for 8-10 minutes, stirring occasionally, until the chicken is cooked through and the vegetables are tender but still crisp.
6. While the chicken and vegetables are cooking, prepare brown rice or cauliflower rice according to your preference.

7. Serve the Chicken Fajita Bowl by layering the cooked rice with the chicken and vegetable mixture.

8. Garnish with your choice of toppings such as salsa, guacamole, sour cream, shredded cheese, lime wedges, and chopped cilantro.

9. Enjoy this delicious and customizable Chicken Fajita Bowl as a wholesome and satisfying meal!

Garlic Turkey Breasts With Lemon

Ingredients:
- 4 turkey breast cutlets
- 4 cloves garlic, minced
- Zest of 1 lemon
- Juice of 1 lemon
- 2 tablespoons olive oil
- 1 teaspoon dried thyme
- 1 teaspoon dried rosemary
- Salt and black pepper to taste
- Fresh parsley for garnish (optional)

Instructions:
1. Preheat the oven to 375°F (190°C).
2. In a small bowl, combine minced garlic, lemon zest, lemon juice, olive oil, dried thyme, dried

rosemary, salt, and black pepper to create the marinade.

3. Place the turkey breast cutlets in a baking dish.

4. Pour the marinade over the turkey, ensuring each cutlet is well coated. Allow it to marinate for at least 15 minutes.

5. Bake in the preheated oven for 20-25 minutes or until the turkey is cooked through and reaches a safe internal temperature.

6. Optionally, broil for an additional 2-3 minutes to achieve a golden brown color on top.

7. Once done, remove from the oven and let the Garlic Turkey Breasts with Lemon rest for a few minutes.

8. Optionally, garnish with fresh parsley for added freshness.

9. Serve the turkey breasts with your favorite side dishes.

10. Enjoy this flavorful and aromatic dish that combines the boldness of garlic with the brightness of lemon!

Chunky Beef and Potato Slow Roast

Ingredients:

- 2 pounds beef stew meat, cut into chunks
- 4 large potatoes, peeled and diced
- 2 carrots, peeled and sliced
- 1 onion, chopped
- 3 cloves garlic, minced
- 2 tablespoons tomato paste
- 1 cup beef broth
- 1 cup red wine (optional)
- 2 tablespoons all-purpose flour
- 2 tablespoons olive oil
- 1 teaspoon dried thyme
- 1 teaspoon dried rosemary
- Salt and black pepper to taste
- Fresh parsley for garnish (optional)

Instructions:

1. Preheat the oven to 325°F (163°C).
2. In a large bowl, toss the beef chunks with flour until they are lightly coated.
3. Heat olive oil in a large oven-safe pot or Dutch oven over medium-high heat. Brown the beef chunks on all sides.

4. Add chopped onion and minced garlic to the pot. Sauté until the onion is softened.

5. Stir in tomato paste and cook for 1-2 minutes to enhance its flavor.

6. Pour in beef broth and red wine (if using), scraping the bottom of the pot to release any browned bits.

7. Add diced potatoes and sliced carrots to the pot. Mix well.

8. Season with dried thyme, dried rosemary, salt, and black pepper. Stir to combine.

9. Cover the pot and transfer it to the preheated oven.

10. Slow roast for 2.5 to 3 hours or until the beef is tender and the flavors have melded.

11. Once done, remove from the oven and let it rest for a few minutes.

12. Optionally, garnish with fresh parsley.

13. Serve the Chunky Beef and Potato Slow Roast as a hearty and comforting meal.

14. Enjoy this classic slow-cooked dish that combines tender beef with flavorful potatoes and carrots!

Spiced Lamb Burgers

Ingredients:

- 1 pound ground lamb
- 1/2 cup breadcrumbs
- 1 small red onion, finely chopped
- 2 cloves garlic, minced
- 1 teaspoon ground cumin
- 1 teaspoon ground coriander
- 1/2 teaspoon paprika
- 1/2 teaspoon ground cinnamon
- 1/4 teaspoon cayenne pepper (adjust to taste)
- Salt and black pepper to taste
- 2 tablespoons fresh mint, chopped
- 2 tablespoons fresh parsley, chopped
- Olive oil for grilling
- Burger buns and your choice of toppings

Instructions:

1. In a large bowl, combine ground lamb, breadcrumbs, chopped red onion, minced garlic, ground cumin, ground coriander, paprika, ground cinnamon, cayenne pepper, salt, and black pepper.

2. Add chopped fresh mint and fresh parsley to the mixture. Mix everything together until well combined.

3. Divide the lamb mixture into equal portions and shape them into burger patties.

4. Preheat a grill or grill pan over medium-high heat. Brush the grates with a bit of olive oil to prevent sticking.

5. Grill the lamb burgers for about 4-5 minutes per side, or until they reach your desired level of doneness.

6. While grilling, toast the burger buns on the grill for a minute or until they are lightly browned.

7. Once done, assemble the Spiced Lamb Burgers on the toasted buns and add your choice of toppings.

8. Serve the lamb burgers immediately.

9. Enjoy these flavorful and spiced lamb burgers, combining the richness of lamb with aromatic spices and fresh herbs!

Meatballs with Ginger

Ingredients:

For the Meatballs:

- 1 pound ground beef or a mixture of beef and pork
- 1/2 cup breadcrumbs
- 1/4 cup milk
- 1/4 cup grated Parmesan cheese
- 1/4 cup chopped fresh parsley
- 1 egg
- 2 cloves garlic, minced
- 1 teaspoon ground ginger
- Salt and black pepper to taste

For the Sauce:

- 1 tablespoon olive oil
- 1 small onion, finely chopped
- 2 cloves garlic, minced
- 1 teaspoon grated ginger
- 1 can (14 oz) crushed tomatoes
- 1 teaspoon soy sauce
- 1 teaspoon honey or maple syrup
- Salt and black pepper to taste
- Fresh cilantro for garnish (optional)

Instructions:

1. Preheat the oven to 400°F (200°C).

2. In a bowl, combine ground beef, breadcrumbs, milk, grated Parmesan cheese, chopped fresh parsley, egg, minced garlic, ground ginger, salt, and black pepper. Mix until well combined.

3. Shape the mixture into meatballs, about 1-1.5 inches in diameter, and place them on a baking sheet lined with parchment paper.

4. Bake the meatballs in the preheated oven for 20-25 minutes, or until they are cooked through and browned.

5. While the meatballs are baking, prepare the sauce. In a skillet, heat olive oil over medium heat.

6. Add finely chopped onion to the skillet and sauté until softened.

7. Stir in minced garlic and grated ginger, cooking for an additional minute until fragrant.

8. Pour in crushed tomatoes, soy sauce, honey or maple syrup, salt, and black pepper. Simmer the sauce for about 10-15 minutes to allow the flavors to meld.

9. Once the meatballs are done baking, transfer them to the skillet with the sauce. Coat the meatballs in the ginger sauce and let them simmer for an additional 5 minutes.

10. Optionally, garnish with fresh cilantro for added freshness.

11. Serve the Meatballs with Ginger over rice, pasta, or with a side of crusty bread.

12. Enjoy these flavorful meatballs with a hint of ginger in a savory and slightly sweet tomato sauce!

Cauliflower Shawarma With Tahini

Ingredients:

For the Cauliflower Shawarma:

- 1 large cauliflower, cut into florets
- 3 tablespoons olive oil
- 1 teaspoon ground cumin
- 1 teaspoon ground coriander
- 1 teaspoon smoked paprika
- 1 teaspoon ground turmeric
- 1/2 teaspoon ground cinnamon
- 1/2 teaspoon cayenne pepper (adjust to taste)
- Salt and black pepper to taste

For the Tahini Sauce:

- 1/2 cup tahini
- 2 tablespoons lemon juice
- 2 tablespoons water
- 1 clove garlic, minced
- 1/2 teaspoon ground cumin
- Salt to taste

For Serving:

- Pita bread or flatbreads
- Sliced cucumbers, tomatoes, and red onions
- Fresh parsley or cilantro for garnish

Instructions:

1. Preheat the oven to 425°F (220°C).
2. In a large bowl, toss cauliflower florets with olive oil, ground cumin, ground coriander, smoked paprika, ground turmeric, ground cinnamon, cayenne pepper, salt, and black pepper until the cauliflower is well coated.
3. Spread the seasoned cauliflower on a baking sheet in a single layer.
4. Roast in the preheated oven for 25-30 minutes or until the cauliflower is golden brown and crisp around the edges, tossing halfway through.

5. While the cauliflower is roasting, prepare the tahini sauce. In a bowl, whisk together tahini, lemon juice, water, minced garlic, ground cumin, and salt until smooth. Adjust the consistency with more water if needed.

6. Once the cauliflower is done, assemble your Cauliflower Shawarma by placing it in pita bread or flatbreads.

7. Top with sliced cucumbers, tomatoes, red onions, and drizzle with the tahini sauce.

8. Optionally, garnish with fresh parsley or cilantro.

9. Serve the Cauliflower Shawarma with Tahini immediately.

10. Enjoy this plant-based twist on shawarma, where the spiced roasted cauliflower meets the creamy tahini sauce for a delightful and satisfying dish!

Green Pesto Pasta

Ingredients:

- 8 oz (about 225g) pasta (spaghetti, fettuccine, or your choice)
- 2 cups fresh basil leaves, packed
- 1/2 cup grated Parmesan cheese

- 1/3 cup pine nuts, toasted
- 2 cloves garlic, peeled
- 1/2 cup extra-virgin olive oil
- Salt and black pepper to taste
- 1/2 cup cherry tomatoes, halved
- Grated Parmesan for serving
- Optional: Extra basil leaves and pine nuts for garnish

Instructions:

1. Cook the pasta according to the package instructions. Reserve a cup of pasta cooking water before draining.
2. In a food processor, combine fresh basil, grated Parmesan, toasted pine nuts, and peeled garlic.
3. Pulse the ingredients until coarsely chopped.
4. With the food processor running, slowly pour in the olive oil in a steady stream until the pesto reaches a smooth consistency.
5. Season the pesto with salt and black pepper to taste. Adjust the seasoning if needed.
6. In a large mixing bowl, toss the cooked pasta with the freshly made pesto. If the pesto is too thick, add some of the reserved pasta cooking water to reach your desired consistency.
7. Gently fold in the halved cherry tomatoes.

8. Serve the Green Pesto Pasta on plates, topped with additional grated Parmesan.
9. Optionally, garnish with extra basil leaves and pine nuts for a decorative touch.
10. Enjoy this vibrant and flavorful Green Pesto Pasta as a quick and delicious meal!

Glazed Tempeh

Ingredients:

- 8 oz (about 225g) tempeh, cut into cubes or strips
- 1/4 cup soy sauce
- 2 tablespoons maple syrup or agave nectar
- 1 tablespoon rice vinegar
- 1 tablespoon sesame oil
- 2 cloves garlic, minced
- 1 teaspoon grated ginger
- 1 tablespoon vegetable oil (for cooking)
- Optional toppings: sesame seeds, chopped green onions

Instructions:

1. In a bowl, whisk together soy sauce, maple syrup or agave nectar, rice vinegar, sesame oil, minced garlic, and grated ginger to create the glaze.

2. Place the tempeh cubes or strips in a shallow dish and pour half of the glaze over them. Allow the tempeh to marinate for at least 15 minutes.

3. Heat vegetable oil in a skillet over medium-high heat.

4. Add the marinated tempeh to the skillet, reserving the marinade for later.

5. Cook the tempeh for 3-4 minutes on each side or until golden brown and slightly crispy.

6. Pour the remaining glaze over the cooking tempeh, allowing it to coat and caramelize the tempeh pieces.

7. Cook for an additional 2-3 minutes, ensuring the glaze thickens and coats the tempeh evenly.

8. Optionally, sprinkle sesame seeds and chopped green onions over the glazed tempeh for added flavor and presentation.

9. Serve the Glazed Tempeh over rice, quinoa, or your favorite grain.

10. Enjoy this sweet and savory glazed tempeh as a protein-rich and flavorful plant-based dish!

Tangy Filets With Sweet Potato Flakes

Ingredients:

For the Tangy Filets:

- 4 white fish filets (such as tilapia or cod)
- 1/4 cup Dijon mustard
- 2 tablespoons honey
- 2 tablespoons apple cider vinegar
- 1 tablespoon olive oil
- 1 teaspoon paprika
- Salt and black pepper to taste

For the Sweet Potato Flakes:

- 2 large sweet potatoes, peeled and spiralized or thinly sliced
- 2 tablespoons olive oil
- 1 teaspoon smoked paprika
- Salt and black pepper to taste

Instructions:

For the Tangy Filets:

1. Preheat the oven to 400°F (200°C). Line a baking sheet with parchment paper.
2. In a bowl, whisk together Dijon mustard, honey, apple cider vinegar, olive oil, paprika, salt, and black pepper.
3. Place the fish filets on the prepared baking sheet.

4. Brush the filets with the tangy mustard mixture, ensuring they are well coated.

5. Bake in the preheated oven for 12-15 minutes or until the fish is cooked through and flakes easily with a fork.

For the Sweet Potato Flakes:

1. In a large bowl, toss sweet potato noodles or slices with olive oil, smoked paprika, salt, and black pepper until evenly coated.

2. Spread the sweet potato mixture on a separate baking sheet.

3. Bake in the preheated oven for 10-15 minutes or until the sweet potato flakes are golden brown and slightly crispy.

4. Serve the Tangy Filets over the Sweet Potato Flakes.

5. Enjoy this tangy and flavorful fish dish paired with the sweetness and crunch of baked sweet potato flakes!

Garlic Turkey Breasts with Lemon

Ingredients:

- 4 turkey breast cutlets
- 4 cloves garlic, minced
- Zest of 1 lemon
- Juice of 1 lemon
- 2 tablespoons olive oil
- 1 teaspoon dried thyme
- 1 teaspoon dried rosemary
- Salt and black pepper to taste
- Fresh parsley for garnish (optional)

Instructions:

1. Preheat the oven to 375°F (190°C).

2. In a small bowl, combine minced garlic, lemon zest, lemon juice, olive oil, dried thyme, dried rosemary, salt, and black pepper to create the marinade.

3. Place the turkey breast cutlets in a baking dish.

4. Pour the marinade over the turkey, ensuring each cutlet is well coated. Allow it to marinate for at least 15 minutes.

5. Bake in the preheated oven for 20-25 minutes or until the turkey is cooked through and reaches a safe internal temperature.

6. Optionally, broil for an additional 2-3 minutes to achieve a golden brown color on top.

7. Once done, remove from the oven and let the Garlic Turkey Breasts with Lemon rest for a few minutes.

8. Optionally, garnish with fresh parsley for added freshness.

9. Serve the turkey breasts with your favorite side dishes.

10. Enjoy this flavorful and aromatic dish that combines the boldness of garlic with the brightness of lemon!

Garlicky Barley and Pinto Beans

Ingredients:

- 1 cup barley, rinsed
- 2 1/2 cups vegetable broth
- 1 cup dried pinto beans, soaked overnight and drained
- 1 onion, finely chopped
- 4 cloves garlic, minced
- 2 tablespoons olive oil
- 1 teaspoon cumin
- 1/2 teaspoon smoked paprika

- Salt and black pepper to taste
- Fresh cilantro for garnish (optional)
- Lime wedges for serving

Instructions:

1. In a large pot, heat olive oil over medium heat. Add chopped onion and sauté until softened.

2. Add minced garlic to the pot and sauté for an additional minute until fragrant.

3. Stir in cumin and smoked paprika, coating the onions and garlic in the spices.

4. Add rinsed barley and soaked pinto beans to the pot. Stir to combine with the aromatic mixture.

5. Pour in vegetable broth and bring the mixture to a boil. Once boiling, reduce the heat to low, cover the pot, and simmer for about 40-45 minutes or until the barley and beans are tender.

6. Season with salt and black pepper to taste. Adjust the seasoning as needed.

7. Optionally, garnish with fresh cilantro for added freshness.

8. Serve the Garlicky Barley and Pinto Beans hot, with lime wedges on the side.

9. Enjoy this wholesome and flavorful dish that combines the nuttiness of barley with the earthy richness of pinto beans and aromatic garlic!

Creamy Broccoli and Sweet Potato Soup

Ingredients:

- 2 cups broccoli florets
- 2 medium-sized sweet potatoes, peeled and diced
- 1 onion, chopped
- 2 cloves garlic, minced
- 4 cups vegetable broth
- 1 cup coconut milk
- 2 tablespoons olive oil
- 1 teaspoon curry powder
- 1/2 teaspoon ground cumin
- Salt and black pepper to taste
- Optional toppings: roasted pumpkin seeds, a drizzle of coconut milk, chopped fresh cilantro

Instructions:

1. In a large pot, heat olive oil over medium heat. Add chopped onion and sauté until translucent.

2. Add minced garlic to the pot and sauté for an additional minute until fragrant.

3. Stir in curry powder and ground cumin, coating the onions and garlic in the spices.

4. Add diced sweet potatoes and broccoli florets to the pot. Mix well with the aromatic mixture.

5. Pour in vegetable broth, covering the vegetables. Bring the mixture to a boil, then reduce the heat to low, cover the pot, and simmer for about 15-20 minutes or until the sweet potatoes are tender.

6. Using an immersion blender, blend the soup until smooth and creamy. Alternatively, transfer the soup to a blender in batches, blending until smooth, and then return it to the pot.

7. Stir in coconut milk, and season the soup with salt and black pepper to taste. Adjust the seasoning as needed.

8. Simmer the soup for an additional 5 minutes to allow the flavors to meld.

9. Serve the Creamy Broccoli and Sweet Potato Soup hot.

10. Optionally, top each bowl with roasted pumpkin seeds, a drizzle of coconut milk, and chopped fresh cilantro for added texture and flavor.

11. Enjoy this velvety and nutritious soup that combines the sweetness of sweet potatoes with the earthy goodness of broccoli!

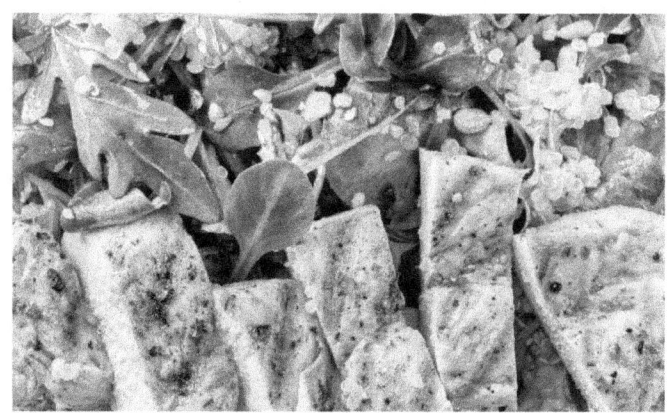

CHAPTER 7: VEGETARIAN DISHES

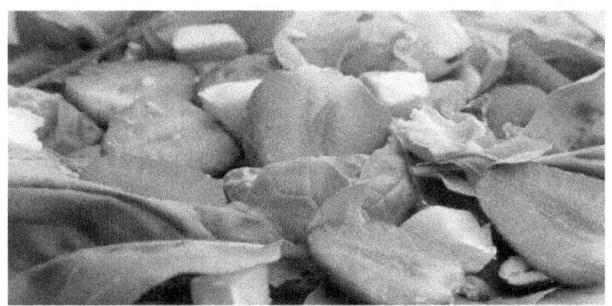

Lentils and Spinach

Ingredients:

- 1 cup dried green or brown lentils, rinsed
- 1 onion, finely chopped
- 3 cloves garlic, minced
- 1 carrot, diced
- 1 celery stalk, diced
- 1 can (14 oz) diced tomatoes
- 4 cups vegetable broth
- 4 cups fresh spinach, washed and chopped
- 1 teaspoon ground cumin
- 1 teaspoon ground coriander
- 1/2 teaspoon smoked paprika

- Salt and black pepper to taste
- 2 tablespoons olive oil
- Lemon wedges for serving (optional)

Instructions:

1. In a large pot, heat olive oil over medium heat. Add chopped onion, diced carrot, and diced celery. Sauté until the vegetables are softened.

2. Add minced garlic to the pot and sauté for an additional minute until fragrant.

3. Stir in rinsed lentils, diced tomatoes (with their juice), ground cumin, ground coriander, smoked paprika, salt, and black pepper.

4. Pour in vegetable broth and bring the mixture to a boil. Once boiling, reduce the heat to low, cover the pot, and simmer for about 25-30 minutes or until the lentils are tender.

5. Stir in chopped spinach and let it wilt into the soup.

6. Adjust the seasoning with additional salt and black pepper if needed.

7. Optionally, squeeze some lemon juice over the Lentils and Spinach for added brightness.

8. Serve the Lentils and Spinach hot.

9. Enjoy this nutritious and flavorful dish that combines the earthiness of lentils with the freshness of spinach!

Salad With Strawberries and Goat Cheese

Ingredients:

- 6 cups mixed salad greens (spinach, arugula, and/or lettuce)
- 1 cup strawberries, hulled and sliced
- 1/2 cup crumbled goat cheese
- 1/2 cup candied pecans or walnuts
- 1/4 cup red onion, thinly sliced
- Balsamic vinaigrette dressing

Instructions:

1. In a large salad bowl, combine the mixed salad greens.
2. Add sliced strawberries, crumbled goat cheese, candied pecans or walnuts, and thinly sliced red onion on top of the greens.
3. Drizzle the salad with balsamic vinaigrette dressing. Start with a small amount and adjust according to your taste.

4. Gently toss the salad ingredients to combine everything evenly.

5. Serve the Salad With Strawberries and Goat Cheese immediately.

6. Enjoy this refreshing and delightful salad that balances the sweetness of strawberries with the tanginess of goat cheese and the crunch of candied nuts!

Vegetable Stew With Mediterranean Spices

Ingredients:

- 2 tablespoons olive oil
- 1 onion, chopped
- 3 cloves garlic, minced
- 1 eggplant, diced
- 2 zucchini, diced
- 1 red bell pepper, diced
- 1 yellow bell pepper, diced
- 1 can (14 oz) diced tomatoes
- 1 can (15 oz) chickpeas, drained and rinsed
- 3 cups vegetable broth
- 1 teaspoon dried oregano
- 1 teaspoon dried thyme

- 1 teaspoon ground cumin
- 1 teaspoon smoked paprika
- Salt and black pepper to taste
- Fresh parsley for garnish

Instructions:

1. In a large pot, heat olive oil over medium heat. Add chopped onion and sauté until softened.

2. Add minced garlic to the pot and sauté for an additional minute until fragrant.

3. Stir in diced eggplant, zucchini, red bell pepper, and yellow bell pepper. Cook for about 5-7 minutes until the vegetables start to soften.

4. Add diced tomatoes, chickpeas, vegetable broth, dried oregano, dried thyme, ground cumin, smoked paprika, salt, and black pepper.

5. Bring the mixture to a boil, then reduce the heat to low, cover the pot, and simmer for about 20-25 minutes or until the vegetables are tender.

6. Adjust the seasoning with additional salt and black pepper if needed.

7. Optionally, garnish the Vegetable Stew With Mediterranean Spices with fresh parsley for added freshness.

8. Serve the vegetable stew hot.

9. Enjoy this flavorful and hearty stew that brings together the vibrant colors and Mediterranean spices!

Soft Red Cabbage With Cranberry

Ingredients:

- 1 medium-sized red cabbage, thinly shredded
- 1 cup fresh or frozen cranberries
- 1/2 cup red onion, thinly sliced
- 1/4 cup apple cider vinegar
- 1/4 cup brown sugar
- 1/4 cup water
- 2 tablespoons olive oil
- 1 teaspoon ground cinnamon
- 1/2 teaspoon ground cloves
- Salt and black pepper to taste
- Orange zest for garnish (optional)

Instructions:

1. In a large pan or skillet, heat olive oil over medium heat. Add thinly sliced red onion and sauté until softened.

2. Add shredded red cabbage to the pan and continue to sauté for about 5 minutes until the cabbage starts to wilt.

3. Stir in cranberries, ground cinnamon, ground cloves, brown sugar, apple cider vinegar, and water.

4. Reduce the heat to low, cover the pan, and let the mixture simmer for 15-20 minutes or until the cabbage is tender and the cranberries have burst.

5. Season the Soft Red Cabbage With Cranberry with salt and black pepper to taste. Adjust the seasoning as needed.

6. Optionally, garnish with orange zest for a citrusy twist.

7. Serve the soft red cabbage hot as a festive and flavorful side dish.

8. Enjoy this vibrant and tangy dish that combines the sweetness of cranberries with the earthiness of red cabbage!

Thai Tofu Broth

Ingredients:
- 1 block firm tofu, cubed
- 4 cups vegetable broth
- 1 can (14 oz) coconut milk
- 1 red bell pepper, thinly sliced
- 1 carrot, julienned

- 1 zucchini, thinly sliced
- 3 cloves garlic, minced
- 1 thumb-sized ginger, grated
- 2 tablespoons soy sauce
- 1 tablespoon red curry paste
- 1 tablespoon lime juice
- 1 tablespoon brown sugar
- 2 tablespoons vegetable oil
- Fresh cilantro for garnish
- Cooked rice noodles or rice for serving

Instructions:

1. In a large pot, heat vegetable oil over medium heat. Add minced garlic and grated ginger, sautéing until fragrant.
2. Stir in red curry paste and cook for an additional minute.
3. Add cubed tofu to the pot and cook for 3-4 minutes, allowing it to brown slightly.
4. Pour in vegetable broth and coconut milk, stirring to combine.
5. Add thinly sliced red bell pepper, julienned carrot, and thinly sliced zucchini to the pot. Simmer for about 10-15 minutes or until the vegetables are tender.

6. In a small bowl, mix soy sauce, lime juice, and brown sugar. Add this mixture to the pot, adjusting the flavors to your liking.

7. Optionally, season the Thai Tofu Broth with salt if needed.

8. Serve the Thai Tofu Broth over cooked rice noodles or rice.

9. Garnish with fresh cilantro for added freshness.

10. Enjoy this flavorful and aromatic Thai-inspired broth with tofu and a variety of colorful vegetables!

Roasted Garlic Lemon Cauliflower

Ingredients:
- 1 head cauliflower, cut into florets
- 4 cloves garlic, minced
- Zest of 1 lemon
- Juice of 1 lemon
- 3 tablespoons olive oil
- 1 teaspoon dried thyme
- Salt and black pepper to taste
- Fresh parsley for garnish (optional)

Instructions:
1. Preheat the oven to 400°F (200°C).

2. In a large mixing bowl, combine cauliflower florets, minced garlic, lemon zest, lemon juice, olive oil, dried thyme, salt, and black pepper. Toss until the cauliflower is well coated.

3. Spread the seasoned cauliflower evenly on a baking sheet lined with parchment paper.

4. Roast in the preheated oven for 25-30 minutes or until the cauliflower is golden brown and tender, tossing halfway through for even cooking.

5. Once done, remove from the oven and transfer the Roasted Garlic Lemon Cauliflower to a serving dish.

6. Optionally, garnish with fresh parsley for added freshness.

7. Serve the cauliflower hot as a flavorful and healthy side dish.

8. Enjoy this Roasted Garlic Lemon Cauliflower with its zesty and savory flavors!

Chickpea Curry

Ingredients:

- 2 cans (15 oz each) chickpeas, drained and rinsed
- 1 onion, finely chopped

- 3 cloves garlic, minced
- 1 thumb-sized ginger, grated
- 1 can (14 oz) diced tomatoes
- 1 can (14 oz) coconut milk
- 1 cup vegetable broth
- 1 bell pepper, diced
- 1 zucchini, diced
- 2 tablespoons curry powder
- 1 teaspoon ground cumin
- 1 teaspoon ground coriander
- 1/2 teaspoon turmeric
- 1/2 teaspoon cayenne pepper (adjust to taste)
- Salt and black pepper to taste
- 2 tablespoons vegetable oil
- Fresh cilantro for garnish
- Cooked basmati rice for serving

Instructions:

1. In a large pan or pot, heat vegetable oil over medium heat. Add chopped onion and sauté until softened.
2. Add minced garlic and grated ginger to the pan, continuing to sauté for an additional minute until fragrant.

3. Stir in curry powder, ground cumin, ground coriander, turmeric, and cayenne pepper, coating the onions, garlic, and ginger in the spices.

4. Add diced bell pepper and zucchini to the pan, cooking for 3-4 minutes until the vegetables start to soften.

5. Pour in diced tomatoes, coconut milk, and vegetable broth. Bring the mixture to a simmer.

6. Add drained and rinsed chickpeas to the pan, stirring to combine.

7. Season the Chickpea Curry with salt and black pepper to taste. Adjust the seasoning as needed.

8. Simmer the curry for about 15-20 minutes, allowing the flavors to meld and the chickpeas to absorb the spices.

9. Optionally, garnish with fresh cilantro for added freshness.

10. Serve the Chickpea Curry over cooked basmati rice.

11. Enjoy this hearty and flavorful curry that combines the protein-rich chickpeas with a variety of aromatic spices!

Parsley Root Veg Stew

Ingredients:

- 3 parsley roots, peeled and diced
- 2 carrots, peeled and diced
- 1 parsnip, peeled and diced
- 1 onion, finely chopped
- 3 cloves garlic, minced
- 2 potatoes, peeled and diced
- 1 leek, sliced (white and light green parts)
- 4 cups vegetable broth
- 1 can (14 oz) diced tomatoes
- 1 tablespoon tomato paste
- 2 bay leaves
- 1 teaspoon dried thyme
- Salt and black pepper to taste
- 2 tablespoons olive oil
- Fresh parsley for garnish

Instructions:

1. In a large pot, heat olive oil over medium heat. Add chopped onion and sauté until softened.

2. Add minced garlic to the pot and sauté for an additional minute until fragrant.

3. Stir in diced parsley roots, carrots, parsnip, potatoes, and sliced leek. Cook for about 5 minutes, allowing the vegetables to slightly brown.
4. Add vegetable broth, diced tomatoes (with their juice), tomato paste, bay leaves, dried thyme, salt, and black pepper. Bring the mixture to a boil.
5. Once boiling, reduce the heat to low, cover the pot, and simmer for about 25-30 minutes or until the vegetables are tender.
6. Adjust the seasoning with additional salt and black pepper if needed.
7. Optionally, garnish the Parsley Root Veg Stew with fresh parsley for added freshness.
8. Serve the vegetable stew hot.
9. Enjoy this hearty and nutritious stew that showcases the earthy flavors of parsley roots, carrots, parsnip, and potatoes!

Sautéed Green Beans

Ingredients:
- 1 lb green beans, trimmed
- 2 tablespoons olive oil
- 2 cloves garlic, minced

- 1 teaspoon lemon zest
- 1 tablespoon lemon juice
- Salt and black pepper to taste
- Optional: Red pepper flakes for a hint of spice
- Optional: Toasted almonds for garnish

Instructions:

1. Bring a pot of water to a boil. Add a pinch of salt and the trimmed green beans. Blanch the green beans for 2-3 minutes until they are bright green but still crisp. Drain and immediately transfer them to a bowl of ice water to stop the cooking process. Drain again and pat dry.

2. In a large skillet, heat olive oil over medium heat. Add minced garlic and sauté for about 1 minute until fragrant.

3. Add the blanched green beans to the skillet. Sauté for 4-5 minutes, stirring occasionally, until the green beans are tender-crisp.

4. Drizzle lemon juice over the green beans and sprinkle lemon zest. Toss to combine.

5. Season the Sautéed Green Beans with salt and black pepper to taste. If you like a bit of heat, add red pepper flakes.

6. Optionally, garnish with toasted almonds for added crunch.

7. Serve the green beans hot as a vibrant and flavorful side dish.

8. Enjoy these Sautéed Green Beans that are simple, fresh, and bursting with citrusy goodness!

Coconut & Pecan Sweet Potatoes

Ingredients:

- 4 medium-sized sweet potatoes, peeled and diced
- 1/2 cup shredded coconut (unsweetened)
- 1/2 cup chopped pecans
- 1/4 cup maple syrup
- 2 tablespoons coconut oil, melted
- 1 teaspoon ground cinnamon
- 1/2 teaspoon ground nutmeg
- 1/4 teaspoon salt
- Optional: Marshmallows for topping

Instructions:

1. Preheat the oven to 375°F (190°C).

2. In a large mixing bowl, combine diced sweet potatoes, shredded coconut, chopped pecans, maple syrup, melted coconut oil, ground cinnamon, ground nutmeg, and salt. Toss until the sweet potatoes are evenly coated.

3. Transfer the mixture to a baking dish, spreading it out in an even layer.

4. Cover the baking dish with aluminum foil and bake in the preheated oven for about 30 minutes.

5. Remove the foil, stir the Coconut & Pecan Sweet Potatoes, and continue baking uncovered for an additional 15-20 minutes or until the sweet potatoes are tender and the edges are caramelized.

6. If desired, in the last 5 minutes of baking, add marshmallows to the top of the sweet potatoes and broil until they are golden brown and toasted.

7. Remove from the oven and let it cool for a few minutes before serving.

8. Serve the Coconut & Pecan Sweet Potatoes as a delicious and comforting side dish.

9. Enjoy the combination of sweet potatoes, coconut, and pecans with warm spices for a delightful twist!

"My digestion is efficient, and I embrace the benefits of my gallbladder-free lifestyle."

"I prioritize self-care through mindful and satisfying eating habits."

CHAPTER 8: SALADS RECIPES

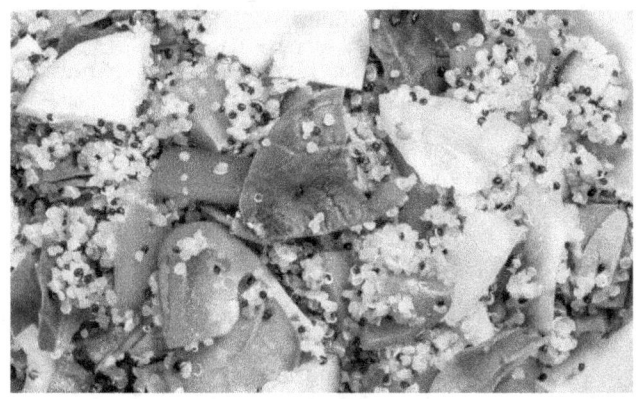

Quinoa Avocado Salad

Ingredients:

- 1 cup quinoa, rinsed
- 2 cups water or vegetable broth
- 2 ripe avocados, diced
- 1 cup cherry tomatoes, halved
- 1/2 cucumber, diced
- 1/4 cup red onion, finely chopped
- 1/4 cup fresh cilantro, chopped
- Juice of 1-2 limes
- 3 tablespoons extra-virgin olive oil
- Salt and black pepper to taste
- Optional: Feta cheese crumbles for garnish

Instructions:

1. In a medium saucepan, combine quinoa and water or vegetable broth. Bring to a boil, then reduce heat to low, cover, and simmer for 15-20 minutes or until the quinoa is cooked and water is absorbed. Fluff with a fork and let it cool.

2. In a large salad bowl, combine the cooked quinoa, diced avocados, halved cherry tomatoes, diced cucumber, chopped red onion, and fresh cilantro.

3. In a small bowl, whisk together lime juice, extra-virgin olive oil, salt, and black pepper to create the dressing.

4. Pour the dressing over the quinoa salad and toss gently to combine, ensuring the ingredients are well coated.

5. Adjust the seasoning if needed, and optionally, garnish the Quinoa Avocado Salad with feta cheese crumbles.

6. Refrigerate the salad for at least 30 minutes to allow the flavors to meld.

7. Serve the chilled salad as a refreshing and nutritious side dish or a light meal.

8. Enjoy this Quinoa Avocado Salad as a wholesome and satisfying dish that celebrates the vibrant colors and flavors of fresh ingredients!

Cantaloupe Salad

Ingredients:

- 1 medium cantaloupe, peeled, seeded, and diced
- 1 cup cherry tomatoes, halved
- 1 cucumber, diced
- 1/4 cup red onion, finely chopped
- 1/4 cup fresh mint leaves, chopped
- 1/4 cup feta cheese, crumbled (optional)
- Juice of 1 lime
- 2 tablespoons extra-virgin olive oil
- Salt and black pepper to taste

Instructions:

1. In a large bowl, combine diced cantaloupe, halved cherry tomatoes, diced cucumber, chopped red onion, and fresh mint leaves.
2. If using, add crumbled feta cheese to the bowl.
3. In a small bowl, whisk together lime juice, extra-virgin olive oil, salt, and black pepper to create the dressing.

4. Pour the dressing over the cantaloupe salad and toss gently to ensure all ingredients are coated.

5. Adjust the seasoning if needed.

6. Refrigerate the Cantaloupe Salad for about 30 minutes before serving to enhance the flavors.

7. Serve the chilled salad as a refreshing and flavorful side dish or a light and healthy snack.

8. Enjoy this Cantaloupe Salad that combines the sweetness of cantaloupe with the crispness of cucumber and the tangy notes of lime!

Lentil Super Salad

Ingredients:
- 1 cup dry green lentils
- 3 cups water or vegetable broth
- 1 cucumber, diced
- 1 bell pepper (any color), diced
- 1 cup cherry tomatoes, halved
- 1/2 red onion, finely chopped
- 1/4 cup fresh parsley, chopped
- 1/4 cup feta cheese, crumbled (optional)
- Juice of 1 lemon
- 3 tablespoons extra-virgin olive oil
- 1 teaspoon Dijon mustard

- 1 clove garlic, minced
- Salt and black pepper to taste
- Optional: Avocado slices for garnish

Instructions:

1. Rinse the green lentils under cold water. In a saucepan, combine lentils and water or vegetable broth. Bring to a boil, then reduce heat to low, cover, and simmer for 20-25 minutes or until the lentils are tender but still firm. Drain any excess liquid and let them cool.

2. In a large salad bowl, combine cooked lentils, diced cucumber, diced bell pepper, halved cherry tomatoes, chopped red onion, and fresh parsley.

3. If using, add crumbled feta cheese to the bowl.

4. In a small bowl, whisk together lemon juice, extra-virgin olive oil, Dijon mustard, minced garlic, salt, and black pepper to create the dressing.

5. Pour the dressing over the Lentil Super Salad and toss gently to ensure all ingredients are coated.

6. Adjust the seasoning if needed.

7. Optionally, garnish the salad with avocado slices.

8. Refrigerate the Lentil Super Salad for at least 30 minutes to allow the flavors to meld.

9. Serve the chilled salad as a hearty and nutritious main dish or a side dish.

10. Enjoy this Lentil Super Salad that packs a punch of protein, fiber, and vibrant flavors!

Quinoa-Black Bean Salad

Ingredients:

- 1 cup quinoa, rinsed
- 2 cups water or vegetable broth
- 1 can (15 oz) black beans, drained and rinsed
- 1 cup corn kernels (fresh, frozen, or canned)
- 1 red bell pepper, diced
- 1/2 red onion, finely chopped
- 1/4 cup fresh cilantro, chopped
- Juice of 2 limes
- 3 tablespoons extra-virgin olive oil
- 1 teaspoon ground cumin
- 1/2 teaspoon chili powder
- Salt and black pepper to taste
- Optional: Avocado slices for garnish

Instructions:

1. In a medium saucepan, combine quinoa and water or vegetable broth. Bring to a boil, then reduce heat to low, cover, and simmer for 15-20 minutes or until the quinoa is cooked and water is absorbed. Fluff with a fork and let it cool.

2. In a large salad bowl, combine the cooked quinoa, drained black beans, corn kernels, diced red bell pepper, chopped red onion, and fresh cilantro.

3. In a small bowl, whisk together lime juice, extra-virgin olive oil, ground cumin, chili powder, salt, and black pepper to create the dressing.

4. Pour the dressing over the Quinoa-Black Bean Salad and toss gently to ensure all ingredients are coated.

5. Adjust the seasoning if needed.

6. Optionally, garnish the salad with avocado slices.

7. Refrigerate the salad for at least 30 minutes before serving to allow the flavors to meld.

8. Serve the chilled salad as a wholesome and protein-packed main dish or a side dish.

9. Enjoy this Quinoa-Black Bean Salad that combines the goodness of quinoa and black beans with vibrant veggies and zesty lime dressing!

Chickpea Salad Wrap

Ingredients:

For the Chickpea Salad:

- 1 can (15 oz) chickpeas, drained and rinsed
- 1/2 cup cucumber, diced
- 1/2 cup cherry tomatoes, halved
- 1/4 cup red onion, finely chopped
- 1/4 cup Kalamata olives, sliced
- 1/4 cup feta cheese, crumbled
- 2 tablespoons fresh parsley, chopped
- Juice of 1 lemon
- 3 tablespoons extra-virgin olive oil
- 1 teaspoon dried oregano
- Salt and black pepper to taste

For the Wrap:

- Whole grain or spinach wraps
- Hummus for spreading
- Fresh spinach leaves

- Optional additional toppings: Sliced cucumber, cherry tomatoes, red onion, feta cheese

Instructions:

For the Chickpea Salad:

1. In a large bowl, combine drained and rinsed chickpeas, diced cucumber, halved cherry tomatoes, chopped red onion, sliced Kalamata olives, crumbled feta cheese, and chopped fresh parsley.

2. In a small bowl, whisk together lemon juice, extra-virgin olive oil, dried oregano, salt, and black pepper to create the dressing.

3. Pour the dressing over the chickpea salad and toss gently to ensure all ingredients are coated.

4. Adjust the seasoning if needed.

For the Wrap:

1. Spread a generous layer of hummus onto each whole grain or spinach wrap.

2. Place a handful of fresh spinach leaves on top of the hummus.

3. Spoon the prepared Chickpea Salad onto the center of each wrap.

4. Optionally, add additional toppings such as sliced cucumber, cherry tomatoes, red onion, and more feta cheese.

5. Fold in the sides of the wrap and then roll it tightly from the bottom, creating a secure wrap.

6. Repeat the process for each wrap.

7. Slice the wraps in half diagonally and serve.

8. Enjoy these Chickpea Salad Wraps as a nutritious and satisfying meal that combines the flavors of the Mediterranean in a convenient wrap form!

Beet Salad

Ingredients:
- 4 medium-sized beets, peeled and diced
- 1/2 cup walnuts, toasted and chopped
- 1/2 cup feta cheese, crumbled
- 1/4 cup red onion, thinly sliced
- 1/4 cup fresh parsley, chopped
- 3 tablespoons balsamic vinegar
- 2 tablespoons extra-virgin olive oil
- 1 teaspoon Dijon mustard
- Salt and black pepper to taste
- Optional: Mixed salad greens for serving

Instructions:

1. Preheat the oven to 400°F (200°C).

2. Place diced beets on a baking sheet, drizzle with olive oil, and sprinkle with salt. Toss to coat evenly.

3. Roast the beets in the preheated oven for about 25-30 minutes or until they are tender. Allow them to cool to room temperature.

4. In a large salad bowl, combine roasted beets, toasted and chopped walnuts, crumbled feta cheese, thinly sliced red onion, and chopped fresh parsley.

5. In a small bowl, whisk together balsamic vinegar, extra-virgin olive oil, Dijon mustard, salt, and black pepper to create the dressing.

6. Pour the dressing over the Beet Salad and toss gently to ensure all ingredients are coated.

7. Adjust the seasoning if needed.

8. Optionally, serve the salad on a bed of mixed salad greens for added freshness and presentation.

9. Enjoy this Beet Salad as a vibrant and nutrient-packed dish that combines the earthiness of beets with the richness of feta and the crunch of walnuts!

Fat Flush & Detox Salad

Ingredients:

- 2 cups kale, finely chopped
- 1 cup red cabbage, thinly sliced
- 1 cup broccoli florets, chopped
- 1 cup cauliflower florets, chopped
- 1 medium carrot, julienned or grated
- 1/2 cup radishes, thinly sliced
- 1/4 cup pumpkin seeds
- 1/4 cup sunflower seeds
- 1/4 cup flaxseeds
- 1/4 cup chia seeds
- 1/4 cup extra-virgin olive oil
- Juice of 1 lemon
- 1 tablespoon apple cider vinegar
- 1 tablespoon Dijon mustard
- 1 clove garlic, minced
- Salt and black pepper to taste
- Optional: Avocado slices for garnish

Instructions:

1. In a large salad bowl, combine finely chopped kale, thinly sliced red cabbage, chopped broccoli florets, chopped cauliflower florets, julienned or grated carrot, and thinly sliced radishes.

2. Add pumpkin seeds, sunflower seeds, flaxseeds, and chia seeds to the bowl.

3. In a small bowl, whisk together extra-virgin olive oil, lemon juice, apple cider vinegar, Dijon mustard, minced garlic, salt, and black pepper to create the dressing.

4. Pour the dressing over the Fat Flush & Detox Salad and toss gently to ensure all ingredients are coated.

5. Adjust the seasoning if needed.

6. Optionally, garnish the salad with avocado slices.

7. Allow the salad to sit for a few minutes before serving to let the flavors meld.

8. Enjoy this Fat Flush & Detox Salad as a nutrient-rich and cleansing dish that provides a variety of vitamins, minerals, and healthy fats!

Greek Salad with Edamame

Ingredients:
- 2 cups cherry tomatoes, halved
- 1 cucumber, diced
- 1 cup Kalamata olives, pitted and sliced
- 1/2 red onion, thinly sliced

- 1 cup feta cheese, crumbled
- 1 cup cooked and shelled edamame
- 1/4 cup fresh parsley, chopped
- 3 tablespoons extra-virgin olive oil
- Juice of 1 lemon
- 1 teaspoon dried oregano
- Salt and black pepper to taste
- Optional: Romaine lettuce leaves for serving

Instructions:

1. In a large salad bowl, combine halved cherry tomatoes, diced cucumber, sliced Kalamata olives, thinly sliced red onion, crumbled feta cheese, cooked and shelled edamame, and chopped fresh parsley.

2. In a small bowl, whisk together extra-virgin olive oil, lemon juice, dried oregano, salt, and black pepper to create the dressing.

3. Pour the dressing over the Greek Salad with Edamame and toss gently to ensure all ingredients are coated.

4. Adjust the seasoning if needed.

5. Optionally, serve the salad on a bed of Romaine lettuce leaves for added freshness and presentation.

6. Allow the salad to sit for a few minutes before serving to let the flavors meld.

7. Enjoy this Greek Salad with Edamame as a protein-packed and flavorful dish that puts a twist on the classic Greek salad!

Low-Carb Fruit Salad

Ingredients:

- 1 cup strawberries, hulled and sliced
- 1 cup blueberries
- 1 cup raspberries
- 1 cup blackberries
- 1 cup diced watermelon (choose a smaller portion due to its natural sugar content)
- 1 cup diced cantaloupe
- 1 cup diced cucumber
- 1 tablespoon fresh mint leaves, chopped
- Juice of 1 lime
- 1 tablespoon low-carb sweetener (e.g., erythritol or stevia), optional

Instructions:

1. In a large bowl, combine sliced strawberries, blueberries, raspberries, blackberries, diced watermelon, diced cantaloupe, and diced cucumber.

2. Sprinkle chopped fresh mint leaves over the fruit.

3. Squeeze the juice of one lime over the fruit. Optionally, add a low-carb sweetener if desired.

4. Gently toss the Low-Carb Fruit Salad to ensure the fruits are evenly coated.

5. Allow the fruit salad to sit in the refrigerator for at least 30 minutes to let the flavors meld.

6. Before serving, give the fruit salad a final gentle toss.

7. Serve the low-carb fruit salad as a refreshing and naturally sweet treat.

8. Enjoy this vibrant Low-Carb Fruit Salad that's rich in antioxidants and vitamins without added sugars!

Cucumber & Avocado Salad

Ingredients:
- 2 cucumbers, thinly sliced
- 2 ripe avocados, diced
- 1/4 cup red onion, finely chopped
- 1/4 cup fresh cilantro, chopped
- Juice of 2 limes
- 3 tablespoons extra-virgin olive oil

- 1 teaspoon honey or agave syrup (optional for sweetness)
- Salt and black pepper to taste
- Optional: Chili flakes for a hint of spice

Instructions:

1. In a large bowl, combine thinly sliced cucumbers, diced avocados, finely chopped red onion, and chopped fresh cilantro.

2. In a small bowl, whisk together lime juice, extra-virgin olive oil, honey or agave syrup (if using), salt, and black pepper to create the dressing.

3. Pour the dressing over the Cucumber & Avocado Salad and toss gently to ensure all ingredients are coated.

4. Adjust the seasoning if needed.

5. Optionally, sprinkle chili flakes over the salad for a hint of spice.

6. Allow the salad to sit for a few minutes before serving to let the flavors meld.

7. Serve the Cucumber & Avocado Salad as a refreshing and creamy side dish or a light and healthy snack.

8. Enjoy this simple and flavorful salad that combines the crispness of cucumber with the creaminess of ripe avocados!

Citrus Lime Tofu Salad

Ingredients:

For the Citrus Lime Tofu:

- 1 block extra-firm tofu, pressed and cubed
- Zest of 1 lime
- Juice of 2 limes
- 2 tablespoons soy sauce
- 1 tablespoon sesame oil
- 1 tablespoon maple syrup or agave nectar
- 1 teaspoon grated ginger
- 1 clove garlic, minced
- Salt and black pepper to taste
- 2 tablespoons vegetable oil for cooking

For the Salad:

- Mixed salad greens (e.g., arugula, spinach, romaine)
- 1 orange, peeled and segmented
- 1 grapefruit, peeled and segmented
- 1/4 cup red onion, thinly sliced
- 1/4 cup almonds, sliced and toasted

- 2 tablespoons fresh cilantro, chopped
- Sesame seeds for garnish

For the Dressing:
- Juice of 1 lime
- 2 tablespoons extra-virgin olive oil
- 1 teaspoon Dijon mustard
- Salt and black pepper to taste

Instructions:

For the Citrus Lime Tofu:

1. In a bowl, combine lime zest, lime juice, soy sauce, sesame oil, maple syrup or agave nectar, grated ginger, minced garlic, salt, and black pepper to create the marinade.

2. Place the cubed tofu in the marinade, ensuring each piece is well coated. Let it marinate for at least 15-20 minutes.

3. Heat vegetable oil in a pan over medium heat. Add the marinated tofu cubes and cook until they are golden brown and crispy on all sides.

4. Remove the tofu from the pan and set aside.

For the Salad:

1. In a large bowl, combine mixed salad greens, orange segments, grapefruit segments, thinly sliced red onion, sliced and toasted almonds, and chopped fresh cilantro.

2. Arrange the cooked Citrus Lime Tofu on top of the salad.

For the Dressing:

1. In a small bowl, whisk together lime juice, extra-virgin olive oil, Dijon mustard, salt, and black pepper to create the dressing.

2. Drizzle the dressing over the Citrus Lime Tofu Salad.

3. Garnish with sesame seeds.

4. Toss the salad gently to combine all the ingredients.

5. Serve immediately and enjoy this refreshing and flavorful Citrus Lime Tofu Salad!

Feta, Kale & Pear Salad

Ingredients:

For the Salad:

- 4 cups kale, stems removed and leaves chopped
- 2 ripe pears, thinly sliced
- 1/2 cup crumbled feta cheese
- 1/4 cup red onion, thinly sliced
- 1/4 cup walnuts, chopped and toasted

For the Dressing:

- 3 tablespoons extra-virgin olive oil

- 2 tablespoons balsamic vinegar
- 1 tablespoon honey
- 1 teaspoon Dijon mustard
- Salt and black pepper to taste

Instructions:

1. In a large bowl, place the chopped kale.
2. In a small bowl, whisk together the dressing ingredients: extra-virgin olive oil, balsamic vinegar, honey, Dijon mustard, salt, and black pepper.
3. Drizzle the dressing over the kale and massage it into the leaves. Allow the kale to marinate for about 5-10 minutes, which helps to soften the leaves.
4. Add the thinly sliced pears, crumbled feta cheese, thinly sliced red onion, and toasted walnuts to the kale.
5. Toss the salad gently to combine all the ingredients and coat them with the dressing.
6. Adjust the seasoning if needed.
7. Serve the Feta, Kale & Pear Salad immediately, and enjoy the delightful combination of flavors and textures!
8. This salad can be a delicious and nutritious side dish or a light meal on its own.

"I am resilient, adapting to life without a gallbladder with grace, strength, and determination."

"Every meal I prepare is an opportunity to enhance my health and well-being."

CHAPTER 9: DESSERTS

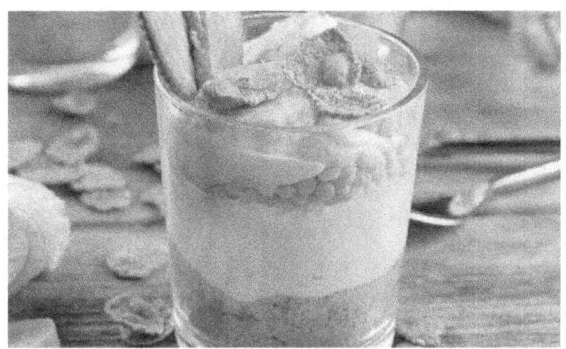

Bagel Bread Pudding

Ingredients:

- 4 bagels (any flavor), cut into bite-sized pieces
- 4 large eggs
- 2 cups whole milk
- 1/2 cup granulated sugar
- 1 teaspoon vanilla extract
- 1/2 teaspoon ground cinnamon
- 1/4 teaspoon salt
- 1/2 cup raisins or dried cranberries (optional)
- 1/2 cup chopped nuts (such as walnuts or pecans), toasted (optional)
- Butter or cooking spray for greasing the baking dish

For the Custard Sauce (Optional):

- 1/2 cup heavy cream
- 1/2 cup whole milk
- 1/4 cup granulated sugar
- 1 teaspoon vanilla extract
- Pinch of salt

Instructions:

1. Preheat the oven to 350°F (175°C). Grease a baking dish with butter or cooking spray.
2. Cut the bagels into bite-sized pieces and spread them evenly in the prepared baking dish.
3. In a mixing bowl, whisk together the eggs, whole milk, granulated sugar, vanilla extract, ground cinnamon, and salt until well combined.
4. Pour the egg mixture over the bagel pieces in the baking dish, making sure all pieces are coated. Allow it to sit for about 10-15 minutes, allowing the bagels to absorb the custard.
5. If desired, sprinkle raisins or dried cranberries and chopped nuts over the bagel mixture.
6. Bake in the preheated oven for approximately 35-40 minutes or until the top is golden brown and the custard is set.

7. While the bread pudding is baking, you can prepare the custard sauce (optional). In a saucepan, combine heavy cream, whole milk, granulated sugar, vanilla extract, and a pinch of salt. Heat over medium-low heat, stirring constantly, until the sugar is dissolved and the mixture is warmed through. Do not bring it to a boil.

8. Once the bread pudding is done, remove it from the oven and let it cool slightly.

9. Serve the bagel bread pudding warm, drizzled with the custard sauce if desired.

10. Enjoy this delightful Bagel Bread Pudding, a creative twist on a classic dessert!

Almond Butter-Quinoa Energy Balls

Ingredients:

- 1 cup cooked quinoa, cooled
- 1/2 cup almond butter
- 1/4 cup honey or maple syrup
- 1/2 cup rolled oats
- 1/4 cup ground flaxseeds
- 1/4 cup shredded coconut (unsweetened)
- 1 teaspoon vanilla extract

- 1/2 teaspoon ground cinnamon
- Pinch of salt
- 1/2 cup chopped almonds (optional, for extra crunch)

Instructions:

1. In a large mixing bowl, combine cooked quinoa, almond butter, honey or maple syrup, rolled oats, ground flaxseeds, shredded coconut, vanilla extract, ground cinnamon, and a pinch of salt.

2. If desired, add chopped almonds to the mixture for extra crunch.

3. Stir the ingredients until well combined. The mixture should be sticky and hold together easily.

4. Place the bowl in the refrigerator for about 30 minutes to make the mixture easier to handle.

5. Once chilled, take small portions of the mixture and roll them into bite-sized balls using your hands. If the mixture is too sticky, you can wet your hands with a little water.

6. Place the energy balls on a parchment paper-lined tray or plate.

7. Once all the mixture is rolled into balls, put the tray or plate in the refrigerator for at least an hour to firm up the energy balls.

8. Store the Almond Butter-Quinoa Energy Balls in an airtight container in the refrigerator. They can be kept for about a week.

9. Enjoy these nutritious and energy-boosting snacks whenever you need a quick pick-me-up during the day!

Chocolate Biscotti with Walnuts

Ingredients:
- 2 cups all-purpose flour
- 1/2 cup unsweetened cocoa powder
- 1 teaspoon baking soda
- 1/4 teaspoon salt
- 1/2 cup unsalted butter, softened
- 1 cup granulated sugar
- 2 large eggs
- 1 teaspoon vanilla extract
- 1 cup walnuts, chopped
- 1 cup semisweet chocolate chips or chunks

Instructions:

1. Preheat your oven to 350°F (175°C). Line a baking sheet with parchment paper.

2. In a medium bowl, whisk together the flour, cocoa powder, baking soda, and salt. Set aside.

3. In a large mixing bowl, cream together the softened butter and granulated sugar until light and fluffy.

4. Add the eggs one at a time, beating well after each addition. Stir in the vanilla extract.

5. Gradually add the dry ingredients to the wet ingredients, mixing until just combined.

6. Fold in the chopped walnuts and semisweet chocolate chips or chunks.

7. Divide the dough in half. On the prepared baking sheet, shape each portion into a log about 12 inches long and 2 inches wide, leaving space between the logs.

8. Bake in the preheated oven for about 25-30 minutes or until the logs are firm to the touch.

9. Remove the logs from the oven and let them cool on the baking sheet for about 15 minutes. Reduce the oven temperature to 325°F (160°C).

10. Transfer the logs to a cutting board and slice them diagonally into 1/2-inch wide pieces.

11. Place the biscotti slices back on the baking sheet, cut side down, and bake for an additional 10-15 minutes or until they become crisp and dry.

12. Allow the chocolate biscotti to cool completely on a wire rack.

13. Optional: Melt additional chocolate and drizzle it over the biscotti for extra decoration.

14. Once fully cooled, store the Chocolate Biscotti with Walnuts in an airtight container.

15. Enjoy these delicious, crunchy biscotti with your favorite hot beverage!

Mini Fruit Pizzas With Pears

Ingredients:

For the Cookie Base:

- 1 cup unsalted butter, softened
- 1 cup granulated sugar
- 1 large egg
- 2 teaspoons vanilla extract
- 3 cups all-purpose flour
- 1/2 teaspoon baking powder

- 1/2 teaspoon salt

For the Cream Cheese Frosting:

- 8 ounces cream cheese, softened
- 1/2 cup unsalted butter, softened
- 2 cups powdered sugar
- 1 teaspoon vanilla extract

For Topping:

- 2 ripe pears, thinly sliced
- 1/4 cup apricot preserves or honey (for glazing the fruit)

Instructions:

For the Cookie Base:

1. Preheat your oven to 350°F (175°C). Line baking sheets with parchment paper.
2. In a large mixing bowl, cream together softened butter and granulated sugar until light and fluffy.
3. Add the egg and vanilla extract, beating until well combined.
4. In a separate bowl, whisk together the flour, baking powder, and salt.
5. Gradually add the dry ingredients to the wet ingredients, mixing until a soft dough forms.

6. Divide the dough into two portions. Roll out each portion between sheets of parchment paper to about 1/4-inch thickness.

7. Using a round cookie cutter, cut out individual cookies and place them on the prepared baking sheets.

8. Bake in the preheated oven for 10-12 minutes or until the edges are lightly golden.

9. Allow the cookies to cool completely on a wire rack.

For the Cream Cheese Frosting:

1. In a bowl, beat together softened cream cheese, softened butter, powdered sugar, and vanilla extract until smooth and creamy.

2. Once the cookies are completely cooled, spread a layer of cream cheese frosting on each cookie.

For Topping:

1. Arrange thinly sliced pears on top of the cream cheese frosting.

2. In a small saucepan, heat apricot preserves until melted. Brush the melted preserves over the sliced pears for a glossy finish.

3. Chill the Mini Fruit Pizzas in the refrigerator for about 30 minutes to allow the frosting to set.

4. Serve and enjoy these delightful Mini Fruit Pizzas with Pears as a sweet and fruity treat!

Papaya and Mint Sorbet

Ingredients:

- 3 cups ripe papaya, peeled, seeded, and cubed
- 1/2 cup fresh mint leaves
- 1/2 cup granulated sugar
- 1/4 cup water
- 2 tablespoons fresh lime juice
- Pinch of salt

Instructions:

1. Place the cubed papaya in a blender or food processor.
2. Add fresh mint leaves to the blender.
3. In a small saucepan, combine granulated sugar and water. Heat over medium heat, stirring until the sugar is completely dissolved. Bring the mixture to a gentle simmer, then remove it from heat.
4. Pour the sugar syrup over the papaya and mint leaves in the blender.
5. Add fresh lime juice and a pinch of salt to the blender.

6. Blend the mixture until smooth and well combined.

7. Taste the sorbet base and adjust the sweetness or lime juice according to your preference.

8. Strain the mixture through a fine-mesh sieve to remove any pulp or mint leaves. This step is optional if you prefer a smoother sorbet.

9. Once strained, transfer the sorbet base to a shallow dish or bowl.

10. Cover the dish with plastic wrap and place it in the freezer for at least 4-6 hours, or until the sorbet is firm.

11. Every hour during the freezing process, use a fork to scrape and fluff the sorbet to prevent it from becoming too icy.

12. Once the Papaya and Mint Sorbet is fully frozen and has a smooth, slushy consistency, it's ready to be served.

13. Scoop the sorbet into bowls or cones, garnish with fresh mint leaves if desired, and enjoy this refreshing and tropical treat!

Pumpkin Cheesecake

Ingredients:

For the Crust:

- 1 1/2 cups graham cracker crumbs
- 1/3 cup unsalted butter, melted
- 2 tablespoons granulated sugar

For the Cheesecake Filling:

- 4 packages (32 ounces) cream cheese, softened
- 1 1/2 cups granulated sugar
- 4 large eggs
- 1 cup canned pumpkin puree
- 1/4 cup all-purpose flour
- 1 teaspoon vanilla extract
- 1 teaspoon ground cinnamon
- 1/2 teaspoon ground nutmeg
- 1/4 teaspoon ground cloves
- 1/4 teaspoon salt

For the Topping:

- 1 cup sour cream
- 2 tablespoons granulated sugar
- 1 teaspoon vanilla extract

Instructions:

For the Crust:

1. Preheat your oven to 325°F (160°C). Grease a 9-inch springform pan.
2. In a bowl, combine graham cracker crumbs, melted butter, and sugar. Press the mixture evenly into the bottom of the prepared springform pan to form the crust.
3. Bake the crust in the preheated oven for 8-10 minutes. Remove from the oven and let it cool while preparing the filling.

For the Cheesecake Filling:

1. In a large mixing bowl, beat the softened cream cheese until smooth and creamy.
2. Add granulated sugar and continue to beat until well combined.
3. Add eggs one at a time, beating well after each addition.
4. Add canned pumpkin puree, flour, vanilla extract, ground cinnamon, ground nutmeg, ground cloves, and salt. Beat until the mixture is smooth and well blended.
5. Pour the pumpkin cheesecake filling over the cooled crust in the springform pan.

6. Tap the pan on the counter to remove any air bubbles.

7. Bake in the preheated oven for 60-70 minutes or until the edges are set, and the center is slightly jiggly.

For the Topping:

1. In a bowl, mix together sour cream, sugar, and vanilla extract.

2. After removing the cheesecake from the oven, spread the sour cream topping evenly over the hot cheesecake.

3. Return the cheesecake to the oven and bake for an additional 10 minutes.

4. Turn off the oven and let the cheesecake cool in the oven with the door ajar for about 1 hour.

5. Remove the cheesecake from the oven and let it cool to room temperature.

6. Refrigerate the pumpkin cheesecake for at least 4 hours or overnight before serving.

7. Once fully chilled, run a knife around the edge of the pan, release the springform, and transfer the cheesecake to a serving plate.

8. Slice and serve your delicious Pumpkin Cheesecake. Optionally, garnish with whipped cream and a sprinkle of ground cinnamon.

Frozen Fantasy

Ingredients:

For the Frozen Fantasy Base:

- 2 cups frozen mixed berries (strawberries, blueberries, raspberries)
- 1 frozen banana, sliced
- 1/2 cup plain Greek yogurt
- 1/4 cup honey or maple syrup
- 1 teaspoon vanilla extract
- 1/2 cup coconut water or any liquid of your choice (adjust as needed)

For the Toppings:

- Fresh berries (for garnish)
- Granola
- Shredded coconut
- Chia seeds
- Mint leaves (optional)

Instructions:

1. In a blender, combine frozen mixed berries, frozen banana slices, Greek yogurt, honey or maple syrup, and vanilla extract.

2. Add coconut water or your preferred liquid to help with blending. Start with a small amount and add more if needed to achieve a smooth consistency.

3. Blend until the mixture is thick and smooth, resembling a soft-serve ice cream texture.

4. Taste the Frozen Fantasy base and adjust sweetness or thickness as desired by adding more honey, maple syrup, or liquid.

5. Once the base is smooth, pour it into bowls or glasses for serving.

6. Garnish the Frozen Fantasy with fresh berries, granola, shredded coconut, chia seeds, and mint leaves if desired.

7. Serve immediately and enjoy this refreshing and healthy Frozen Fantasy as a delightful treat.

Ribbon Cakes

Ingredients:

For the Cake Batter:

- 2 1/2 cups all-purpose flour
- 2 1/2 teaspoons baking powder
- 1/2 teaspoon salt
- 1 cup unsalted butter, softened
- 2 cups granulated sugar
- 4 large eggs
- 1 teaspoon vanilla extract
- 1 cup whole milk

For the Chocolate Ribbon:

- 1/2 cup unsweetened cocoa powder
- 1/4 cup granulated sugar
- 1/4 cup whole milk
- 1/4 cup unsalted butter, melted

For the Vanilla Ribbon:

- 1/4 cup all-purpose flour
- 1/4 cup granulated sugar
- 1/4 cup unsalted butter, melted
- 1 teaspoon vanilla extract

Instructions:

1. Preheat your oven to 350°F (175°C). Grease and flour a Bundt pan.

2. In a medium bowl, whisk together flour, baking powder, and salt. Set aside.

3. In a large mixing bowl, cream together softened butter and granulated sugar until light and fluffy.

4. Add eggs one at a time, beating well after each addition. Stir in vanilla extract.

5. Gradually add the dry ingredients to the wet ingredients, alternating with the cup of whole milk. Begin and end with the dry ingredients, mixing until just combined.

6. Divide the cake batter into three equal portions. Leave one portion as is.

7. For the Chocolate Ribbon: In a separate bowl, whisk together cocoa powder, sugar, milk, and melted butter until smooth. Add this chocolate mixture to one portion of the cake batter, mixing until well combined.

8. For the Vanilla Ribbon: In another bowl, mix together flour, sugar, melted butter, and vanilla extract. Add this mixture to the second portion of the cake batter, stirring until well combined.

9. Leave the third portion of the batter plain.

10. Spoon the three batters alternately into the prepared Bundt pan, creating a layered effect.

11. Use a knife or skewer to gently swirl the batters together, creating a marbled pattern.

12. Bake in the preheated oven for 50-60 minutes or until a toothpick inserted into the center comes out clean.

13. Allow the ribbon cake to cool in the pan for about 15 minutes before transferring it to a wire rack to cool completely.

14. Once cooled, slice and serve this delightful Ribbon Cake with your favorite coffee or tea.

Chocolate Beet Cake

Ingredients:

For the Cake:

- 2 cups cooked and grated beets (about 3-4 medium-sized beets)
- 1 3/4 cups all-purpose flour
- 1/2 cup unsweetened cocoa powder
- 1 1/2 teaspoons baking powder
- 1/2 teaspoon baking soda
- 1/2 teaspoon salt
- 1 1/4 cups granulated sugar
- 1/2 cup vegetable oil
- 3 large eggs
- 1 teaspoon vanilla extract
- 1/2 cup buttermilk

For the Chocolate Ganache (Optional):

- 1/2 cup heavy cream
- 1 cup semi-sweet chocolate chips

Instructions:

1. Preheat your oven to 350°F (175°C). Grease and flour two 9-inch round cake pans.

2. In a medium bowl, whisk together flour, cocoa powder, baking powder, baking soda, and salt. Set aside.

3. In a large mixing bowl, combine grated beets, granulated sugar, vegetable oil, eggs, and vanilla extract. Mix until well combined.

4. Gradually add the dry ingredients to the wet ingredients, alternating with buttermilk. Begin and end with the dry ingredients, mixing until just combined.

5. Divide the batter evenly between the prepared cake pans.

6. Bake in the preheated oven for 25-30 minutes or until a toothpick inserted into the center comes out clean.

7. Allow the cakes to cool in the pans for 10 minutes before transferring them to a wire rack to cool completely.

8. For the Chocolate Ganache (Optional): Heat the heavy cream in a small saucepan until it begins to simmer. Remove from heat and pour it over the chocolate chips in a heatproof bowl. Let it sit for a minute, then stir until smooth. Let the ganache cool slightly before pouring it over the cake.

9. Once the cakes are cooled, you can optionally spread a layer of chocolate ganache between the cake layers and over the top.

10. Slice and serve this rich and moist Chocolate Beet Cake. Enjoy the unique and delicious combination of chocolate and beets!

Strawberry Pie

Ingredients:

For the Pie Crust:

- 1 1/4 cups all-purpose flour
- 1/2 cup unsalted butter, cold and cut into small cubes
- 1/4 cup granulated sugar
- 1/4 teaspoon salt
- 2-3 tablespoons ice water

For the Strawberry Filling:

- 4 cups fresh strawberries, hulled and halved
- 1 cup granulated sugar
- 3 tablespoons cornstarch
- 1/2 teaspoon lemon zest
- 1 tablespoon fresh lemon juice

For the Whipped Cream (Optional):

- 1 cup heavy cream
- 2 tablespoons powdered sugar
- 1 teaspoon vanilla extract

Instructions:

For the Pie Crust:

1. In a food processor, combine flour, cold butter, sugar, and salt. Pulse until the mixture resembles coarse crumbs.
2. Gradually add ice water, one tablespoon at a time, and pulse until the dough comes together.
3. Turn the dough out onto a lightly floured surface and knead it gently into a disk. Wrap it in plastic wrap and refrigerate for at least 1 hour.
4. Preheat your oven to 375°F (190°C).
5. Roll out the chilled dough on a floured surface to fit a 9-inch pie dish.

6. Transfer the dough to the pie dish, trim any excess, and crimp the edges. Prick the bottom of the crust with a fork.

7. Line the crust with parchment paper and fill it with pie weights or dried beans. Bake for about 15 minutes, then remove the parchment paper and weights. Bake for an additional 10-12 minutes or until the crust is golden brown. Allow it to cool completely.

For the Strawberry Filling:

1. In a saucepan, combine sugar and cornstarch. Gradually stir in fresh lemon juice and lemon zest.

2. Cook over medium heat, stirring constantly until the mixture thickens and becomes translucent.

3. Remove the saucepan from heat and let the mixture cool slightly.

4. In a large bowl, gently toss the halved strawberries with the slightly cooled sugar mixture until the berries are well coated.

5. Pour the strawberry filling into the cooled pie crust.

For the Whipped Cream (Optional):

1. In a chilled bowl, whip the heavy cream until soft peaks form.

2. Add powdered sugar and vanilla extract. Continue whipping until stiff peaks form.

3. Dollop the whipped cream over the strawberry filling or serve it on the side when serving individual slices.

4. Refrigerate the Strawberry Pie for at least 3-4 hours before serving to allow the filling to set.

5. Slice and serve this refreshing Strawberry Pie, optionally topped with a dollop of whipped cream.

Pineapple Smoothie

Ingredients:

- 2 cups fresh pineapple chunks (frozen for a thicker smoothie)
- 1 ripe banana
- 1 cup Greek yogurt (vanilla or plain)
- 1/2 cup coconut milk or any milk of your choice
- 1 tablespoon honey or maple syrup (optional, depending on sweetness preference)
- Ice cubes (optional)

Instructions:

1. Peel and chop the fresh pineapple into chunks. If you prefer a colder and thicker smoothie, you can use frozen pineapple chunks.

2. Peel the ripe banana and break it into smaller pieces.

3. In a blender, combine the fresh pineapple chunks, banana pieces, Greek yogurt, coconut milk, and honey (if using).

4. Optional: Add ice cubes for a colder and icier texture.

5. Blend the ingredients on high speed until the mixture is smooth and creamy.

6. Taste the smoothie and adjust the sweetness by adding more honey or maple syrup if needed.

7. Pour the pineapple smoothie into glasses and serve immediately.

8. Garnish with additional pineapple slices or a wedge for presentation, if desired.

Chocolate Cookies without Flour

Ingredients:

- 2 1/2 cups powdered sugar
- 1/2 cup unsweetened cocoa powder

- 1/4 teaspoon salt
- 3 large egg whites, at room temperature
- 1 tablespoon vanilla extract
- 1 cup semisweet chocolate chips

Instructions:

1. Preheat your oven to 350°F (175°C). Line a baking sheet with parchment paper.

2. In a large bowl, whisk together powdered sugar, cocoa powder, and salt until well combined.

3. Add the room temperature egg whites and vanilla extract to the dry ingredients. Mix until the batter is smooth and glossy.

4. Gently fold in the semisweet chocolate chips, distributing them evenly throughout the batter.

5. Drop rounded tablespoons of batter onto the prepared baking sheet, leaving enough space between each cookie.

6. Bake in the preheated oven for 10-12 minutes or until the tops are glossy and set.

7. Allow the chocolate cookies to cool on the baking sheet for a few minutes before transferring them to a wire rack to cool completely.

8. Once cooled, the cookies will have a soft and chewy texture.
9. Store the flourless chocolate cookies in an airtight container at room temperature.

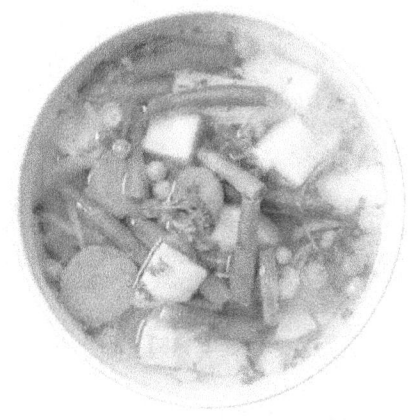

"Every recipe is a step towards a thriving, gallbladder-free life."

"I appreciate the journey of discovering and enjoying new, healthy foods."

CHAPTER 10: SMOOTHIES AND DRINKS

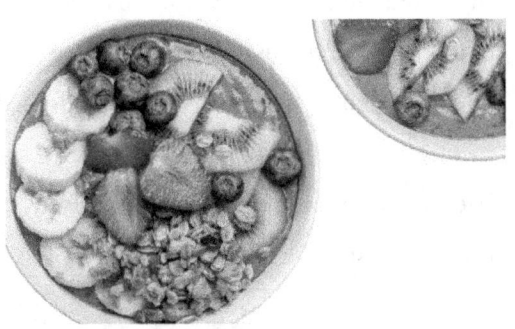

Acai Berry Smoothie

Ingredients:

- 1 packet frozen unsweetened acai berry puree
- 1/2 cup frozen mixed berries (such as blueberries, strawberries, raspberries)
- 1 banana, peeled and sliced
- 1/2 cup plain Greek yogurt
- 1/2 cup almond milk (or any milk of your choice)
- 1 tablespoon honey or maple syrup (optional, depending on sweetness preference)
- Toppings: granola, sliced banana, shredded coconut, chia seeds (optional)

Instructions:

1. Run the frozen acai berry packet under warm water for a few seconds to break it into chunks.

2. In a blender, combine the thawed acai berry chunks, frozen mixed berries, sliced banana, Greek yogurt, almond milk, and honey (if using).

3. Blend the ingredients on high speed until the mixture is smooth and creamy.

4. Taste the smoothie and adjust sweetness by adding more honey if needed.

5. Pour the acai berry smoothie into a bowl.

6. Optionally, top the smoothie with granola, sliced banana, shredded coconut, or chia seeds for added texture and nutrition.

7. Serve immediately and enjoy this vibrant and nutritious Acai Berry Smoothie Bowl!

Watermelon Smoothie

Ingredients:

- 2 cups fresh watermelon, seedless and cubed
- 1 cup frozen strawberries
- 1/2 cup plain Greek yogurt

- 1 tablespoon honey or maple syrup (optional, depending on sweetness preference)
- 1 cup ice cubes
- Mint leaves for garnish (optional)

Instructions:

1. Ensure the watermelon is seedless and cut it into small cubes.
2. In a blender, combine the fresh watermelon cubes, frozen strawberries, Greek yogurt, honey (if using), and ice cubes.
3. Blend the ingredients on high speed until the mixture is smooth and slushy.
4. Taste the smoothie and adjust sweetness by adding more honey if needed.
5. Pour the watermelon smoothie into glasses.
6. Optionally, garnish with mint leaves for a refreshing touch.
7. Serve immediately and enjoy this hydrating and delicious Watermelon Smoothie!

Mango Ginger Smoothie

Ingredients:

- 1 1/2 cups frozen mango chunks
- 1 banana, peeled

- 1/2 cup plain Greek yogurt
- 1 cup coconut water (or regular water)
- 1 tablespoon fresh ginger, peeled and grated
- 1 tablespoon honey or maple syrup (optional, depending on sweetness preference)
- Ice cubes (optional)

Instructions:

1. Peel and grate the fresh ginger.
2. In a blender, combine the frozen mango chunks, peeled banana, Greek yogurt, grated ginger, coconut water, and honey (if using).
3. Blend the ingredients on high speed until the mixture is smooth and creamy.
4. Taste the smoothie and adjust sweetness by adding more honey if needed.
5. If you prefer a colder and icier smoothie, you can add ice cubes at this point and blend again.
6. Pour the mango ginger smoothie into glasses.
7. Serve immediately and enjoy this flavorful and refreshing Mango Ginger Smoothie!

Pomegranate Blackberry Smoothie

Ingredients:

- 1 cup fresh blackberries
- 1/2 cup pomegranate seeds (from about 1 medium pomegranate)
- 1 banana, peeled
- 1/2 cup plain Greek yogurt
- 1 cup pomegranate juice
- 1 tablespoon honey or maple syrup (optional, depending on sweetness preference)
- Ice cubes (optional)

Instructions:

1. Extract the seeds from the pomegranate. Cut the pomegranate in half and hold each half over a bowl, seeds facing down. Tap the back with a wooden spoon to release the seeds. Collect 1/2 cup of seeds.

2. In a blender, combine the fresh blackberries, pomegranate seeds, peeled banana, Greek yogurt, pomegranate juice, and honey (if using).

3. Blend the ingredients on high speed until the mixture is smooth and well combined.

4. Taste the smoothie and adjust sweetness by adding more honey if needed.

5. If you prefer a colder and icier smoothie, you can add ice cubes at this point and blend again.

6. Pour the pomegranate blackberry smoothie into glasses.

7. Serve immediately and enjoy this vibrant and antioxidant-rich Pomegranate Blackberry Smoothie!

Kiwi Strawberry Banana Smoothie

Ingredients:

- 2 ripe kiwis, peeled and sliced
- 1 cup fresh strawberries, hulled
- 1 banana, peeled
- 1/2 cup plain Greek yogurt
- 1 cup orange juice
- 1 tablespoon honey or maple syrup (optional, depending on sweetness preference)
- Ice cubes (optional)

Instructions:

1. Peel and slice the ripe kiwis.
2. Hull the fresh strawberries.
3. In a blender, combine the sliced kiwis, fresh strawberries, peeled banana, Greek yogurt, orange juice, and honey (if using).

4. Blend the ingredients on high speed until the mixture is smooth and well combined.

5. Taste the smoothie and adjust sweetness by adding more honey if needed.

6. If you prefer a colder and icier smoothie, you can add ice cubes at this point and blend again.

7. Pour the kiwi strawberry banana smoothie into glasses.

8. Serve immediately and enjoy this refreshing and vitamin-packed Kiwi Strawberry Banana Smoothie!

Berry Mint Smoothie

Ingredients:

- 1 cup mixed berries (strawberries, blueberries, raspberries)
- 1 banana, peeled
- 1/2 cup plain Greek yogurt
- 1 cup almond milk (or any milk of your choice)
- 1 tablespoon fresh mint leaves
- 1 tablespoon honey or maple syrup (optional, depending on sweetness preference)
- Ice cubes (optional)

Instructions:

1. In a blender, combine the mixed berries, peeled banana, Greek yogurt, almond milk, fresh mint leaves, and honey (if using).

2. Blend the ingredients on high speed until the mixture is smooth and well combined.

3. Taste the smoothie and adjust sweetness by adding more honey if needed.

4. If you prefer a colder and icier smoothie, you can add ice cubes at this point and blend again.

5. Pour the berry mint smoothie into glasses.

6. Optionally, garnish with a few extra mint leaves for a refreshing touch.

7. Serve immediately and enjoy this delightful and antioxidant-rich Berry Mint Smoothie!

Cranberry Ginger Smoothie

Ingredients:

- 1 cup fresh or frozen cranberries
- 1 banana, peeled
- 1/2 cup plain Greek yogurt
- 1 cup orange juice
- 1 tablespoon fresh ginger, peeled and grated

- 1 tablespoon honey or maple syrup (optional, depending on sweetness preference)
- Ice cubes (optional)

Instructions:

1. If using fresh cranberries, rinse them thoroughly. If using frozen cranberries, allow them to thaw slightly.
2. Peel and grate the fresh ginger.
3. In a blender, combine the cranberries, peeled banana, Greek yogurt, orange juice, grated ginger, and honey (if using).
4. Blend the ingredients on high speed until the mixture is smooth and well combined.
5. Taste the smoothie and adjust sweetness by adding more honey if needed.
6. If you prefer a colder and icier smoothie, you can add ice cubes at this point and blend again.
7. Pour the cranberry ginger smoothie into glasses.
8. Serve immediately and enjoy this tangy and invigorating Cranberry Ginger Smoothie!

Banana Protein Smoothie

Ingredients:

- 1 banana, peeled
- 1/2 cup plain Greek yogurt
- 1 cup almond milk (or any milk of your choice)

- 1 scoop protein powder (vanilla or your preferred flavor)
- 1 tablespoon almond butter or peanut butter
- 1 tablespoon chia seeds (optional)
- 1 tablespoon honey or maple syrup (optional, depending on sweetness preference)
- Ice cubes (optional)

Instructions:

1. In a blender, combine the peeled banana, plain Greek yogurt, almond milk, protein powder, almond butter (or peanut butter), chia seeds (if using), and honey (if using).
2. Blend the ingredients on high speed until the mixture is smooth and well combined.
3. Taste the smoothie and adjust sweetness by adding more honey if needed.
4. If you prefer a colder and icier smoothie, you can add ice cubes at this point and blend again.
5. Pour the banana protein smoothie into glasses.
6. Optionally, garnish with a sprinkle of chia seeds or a slice of banana for presentation.
7. Serve immediately and enjoy this protein-packed and energizing Banana Protein Smoothie!

Banana Cauliflower Smoothie

Ingredients:

- 1 banana, peeled
- 1/2 cup steamed cauliflower florets
- 1/2 cup plain Greek yogurt
- 1 cup almond milk (or any milk of your choice)
- 1 tablespoon almond butter or peanut butter
- 1 tablespoon honey or maple syrup (optional, depending on sweetness preference)
- Ice cubes (optional)

Instructions:

1. Steam cauliflower florets until they are tender. Allow them to cool before using.
2. In a blender, combine the peeled banana, steamed cauliflower, plain Greek yogurt, almond milk, almond butter (or peanut butter), and honey (if using).
3. Blend the ingredients on high speed until the mixture is smooth and well combined.
4. Taste the smoothie and adjust sweetness by adding more honey if needed.
5. If you prefer a colder and icier smoothie, you can add ice cubes at this point and blend again.

6. Pour the banana cauliflower smoothie into glasses.

7. Optionally, garnish with a sprinkle of cinnamon or a few chopped nuts for added flavor and texture.

8. Serve immediately and enjoy this unique and nutrient-rich Banana Cauliflower Smoothie!

Pineapple Smoothie

Ingredients:

- 1 cup fresh pineapple chunks (or frozen for a colder smoothie)
- 1 banana, peeled
- 1/2 cup plain Greek yogurt
- 1 cup coconut water (or any liquid of your choice)
- 1 tablespoon honey or maple syrup (optional, depending on sweetness preference)
- Ice cubes (optional)

Instructions:

1. If using fresh pineapple, peel and chop it into chunks. If using frozen pineapple, ensure it's thawed slightly.

2. In a blender, combine the pineapple chunks, peeled banana, plain Greek yogurt, coconut water, and honey (if using).

3. Blend the ingredients on high speed until the mixture is smooth and well combined.

4. Taste the smoothie and adjust sweetness by adding more honey if needed.

5. If you prefer a colder and icier smoothie, you can add ice cubes at this point and blend again.

6. Pour the pineapple smoothie into glasses.

7. Optionally, garnish with a slice of pineapple or a sprinkle of shredded coconut for a tropical touch.

8. Serve immediately and enjoy this refreshing and vitamin-packed Pineapple Smoothie!

Strawberry Raspberry Smoothie

Ingredients:
- 1 cup fresh strawberries, hulled
- 1/2 cup fresh raspberries
- 1 banana, peeled
- 1/2 cup plain Greek yogurt
- 1 cup almond milk (or any milk of your choice)
- 1 tablespoon honey or maple syrup (optional, depending on sweetness preference)

- Ice cubes (optional)

Instructions:

1. Hull the fresh strawberries.

2. In a blender, combine the hulled strawberries, fresh raspberries, peeled banana, plain Greek yogurt, almond milk, and honey (if using).

3. Blend the ingredients on high speed until the mixture is smooth and well combined.

4. Taste the smoothie and adjust sweetness by adding more honey if needed.

5. If you prefer a colder and icier smoothie, you can add ice cubes at this point and blend again.

6. Pour the strawberry raspberry smoothie into glasses.

7. Optionally, garnish with a few whole raspberries or a sliced strawberry for presentation.

8. Serve immediately and enjoy this vibrant and antioxidant-rich Strawberry Raspberry Smoothie!

CHAPTER 11: SOUP RECIPES

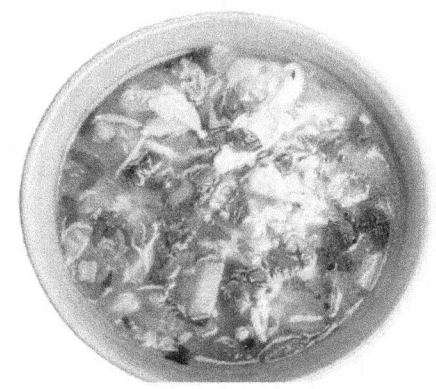

Lentil and Veggie Soup

Ingredients:

- 1 cup dried lentils, rinsed and drained
- 1 onion, finely chopped
- 2 carrots, peeled and diced
- 2 celery stalks, diced
- 3 cloves garlic, minced
- 1 can (14 oz) diced tomatoes
- 6 cups vegetable broth
- 1 teaspoon ground cumin
- 1 teaspoon ground coriander
- 1/2 teaspoon smoked paprika
- 1 bay leaf

- Salt and pepper to taste
- 2 tablespoons olive oil
- Fresh parsley, chopped (for garnish)

Instructions:

1. Heat olive oil in a large pot over medium heat. Add chopped onion, carrots, and celery. Sauté until the vegetables are softened, about 5 minutes.
2. Add minced garlic to the pot and cook for an additional minute until fragrant.
3. Stir in ground cumin, ground coriander, and smoked paprika. Cook for 1-2 minutes to toast the spices.
4. Pour in the rinsed lentils, diced tomatoes (with their juice), and vegetable broth. Add the bay leaf. Bring the soup to a boil, then reduce the heat to low and let it simmer, covered, for about 25-30 minutes or until the lentils are tender.
5. Season the soup with salt and pepper to taste. Adjust the seasoning as needed.
6. Before serving, remove the bay leaf and discard it.
7. Ladle the soup into bowls and garnish with fresh chopped parsley.

Green Chicken Enchilada Soup

Ingredients:

- 1 pound boneless, skinless chicken breasts, cooked and shredded
- 1 tablespoon olive oil
- 1 onion, finely chopped
- 2 cloves garlic, minced
- 1 can (10 oz) green enchilada sauce
- 1 can (4 oz) diced green chilies
- 4 cups chicken broth
- 1 teaspoon ground cumin
- 1 teaspoon chili powder
- 1/2 teaspoon dried oregano
- Salt and pepper to taste
- 1 can (15 oz) white beans, drained and rinsed
- 1 cup frozen corn kernels
- 1 cup shredded Monterey Jack cheese
- Fresh cilantro, chopped (for garnish)
- Lime wedges (for serving)

Instructions:

1. In a large pot, heat olive oil over medium heat. Add chopped onion and cook until softened, about 3-4 minutes.

2. Add minced garlic to the pot and cook for an additional minute until fragrant.

3. Stir in the shredded cooked chicken, green enchilada sauce, diced green chilies, chicken broth, ground cumin, chili powder, dried oregano, salt, and pepper. Bring the mixture to a simmer.

4. Add drained white beans and frozen corn to the pot. Let the soup simmer for another 10-15 minutes, allowing the flavors to meld.

5. Taste the soup and adjust the seasoning if necessary.

6. Just before serving, stir in the shredded Monterey Jack cheese until melted and well combined.

7. Ladle the Green Chicken Enchilada Soup into bowls. Garnish with fresh chopped cilantro.

8. Serve with lime wedges on the side for squeezing over the soup.

Rice and Chicken Soup

Ingredients:
- 1 cup cooked chicken, shredded or diced
- 1 cup cooked rice

- 1 tablespoon olive oil
- 1 onion, finely chopped
- 2 carrots, peeled and diced
- 2 celery stalks, diced
- 3 cloves garlic, minced
- 6 cups chicken broth
- 1 bay leaf
- 1 teaspoon dried thyme
- Salt and pepper to taste
- Fresh parsley, chopped (for garnish)
- Lemon wedges (optional, for serving)

Instructions:

1. In a large pot, heat olive oil over medium heat. Add chopped onion, carrots, and celery. Sauté until the vegetables are softened, about 5 minutes.

2. Add minced garlic to the pot and cook for an additional minute until fragrant.

3. Pour in the chicken broth, add the bay leaf and dried thyme. Bring the mixture to a boil, then reduce the heat to low and let it simmer for about 10-15 minutes to allow the flavors to meld.

4. Add the cooked chicken and rice to the pot. Simmer for an additional 5-10 minutes until the soup is heated through.

5. Season the soup with salt and pepper to taste. Adjust the seasoning as needed.

6. Before serving, remove the bay leaf and discard it.

7. Ladle the Rice and Chicken Soup into bowls. Garnish with fresh chopped parsley.

8. If desired, serve with lemon wedges on the side for a burst of citrus flavor.

Kale Soup

Ingredients:

- 1 bunch kale, stems removed and leaves chopped
- 1 onion, finely chopped
- 2 carrots, peeled and diced
- 2 celery stalks, diced
- 3 cloves garlic, minced
- 1 potato, peeled and diced
- 6 cups vegetable or chicken broth
- 1 can (14 oz) diced tomatoes

- 1 can (15 oz) cannellini beans, drained and rinsed
- 1 teaspoon dried thyme
- 1 teaspoon dried rosemary
- Salt and pepper to taste
- 2 tablespoons olive oil
- Grated Parmesan cheese (for serving)

Instructions:

1. In a large pot, heat olive oil over medium heat. Add chopped onion, carrots, celery, and garlic. Sauté until the vegetables are softened, about 5 minutes.

2. Add diced potatoes to the pot and continue cooking for another 3-4 minutes.

3. Pour in the vegetable or chicken broth, diced tomatoes (with their juice), and drained cannellini beans. Bring the soup to a boil, then reduce the heat to low and let it simmer, covered, for about 15-20 minutes or until the vegetables are tender.

4. Add chopped kale to the pot and simmer for an additional 5-10 minutes until the kale is wilted.

5. Season the soup with dried thyme, dried rosemary, salt, and pepper to taste. Adjust the seasoning as needed.
6. Before serving, ladle the Kale Soup into bowls.
7. Optionally, sprinkle each serving with grated Parmesan cheese.

Creamy Broccoli and Sweet Potato Soup

Ingredients:
- 2 cups broccoli florets
- 1 large sweet potato, peeled and diced
- 1 onion, finely chopped
- 2 cloves garlic, minced
- 4 cups vegetable or chicken broth
- 1 cup milk (or non-dairy milk for a vegan option)
- 2 tablespoons butter (or olive oil for a vegan option)
- 2 tablespoons all-purpose flour (or a gluten-free alternative)
- 1/2 teaspoon ground nutmeg
- Salt and pepper to taste

- 1/2 cup heavy cream (or coconut cream for a vegan option)
- Chopped chives or parsley (for garnish)

Instructions:

1. In a large pot, melt butter (or heat olive oil) over medium heat. Add chopped onion and cook until softened, about 3-4 minutes.

2. Add minced garlic to the pot and cook for an additional minute until fragrant.

3. Sprinkle the flour over the onion and garlic mixture, stirring constantly to create a roux. Cook for 2-3 minutes to eliminate the raw flour taste.

4. Slowly pour in the vegetable or chicken broth, stirring continuously to avoid lumps. Bring the mixture to a gentle boil.

5. Add diced sweet potato to the pot and simmer for about 10-15 minutes or until the sweet potato is tender.

6. Stir in broccoli florets and continue simmering for an additional 5-7 minutes until the broccoli is cooked but still vibrant green.

7. Use an immersion blender to puree the soup until smooth. If you don't have an immersion blender, transfer the soup in batches to a blender and blend until smooth, then return it to the pot.

8. Stir in milk, ground nutmeg, salt, and pepper. Allow the soup to simmer for another 5 minutes.

9. Reduce heat to low and stir in heavy cream (or coconut cream for a vegan option). Adjust the seasoning as needed.

10. Ladle the Creamy Broccoli and Sweet Potato Soup into bowls. Garnish with chopped chives or parsley.

Fresh Kale Garlic Soup

Ingredients:

- 1 bunch fresh kale, stems removed and leaves chopped
- 1 onion, finely chopped
- 4 cloves garlic, minced
- 1 large potato, peeled and diced
- 6 cups vegetable or chicken broth
- 2 tablespoons olive oil
- 1 teaspoon dried thyme
- 1/2 teaspoon red pepper flakes (optional, for a bit of heat)
- Salt and pepper to taste
- Grated Parmesan cheese (for serving)
- Crusty bread (optional, for serving)

Instructions:

1. In a large pot, heat olive oil over medium heat. Add chopped onion and cook until softened, about 3-4 minutes.

2. Add minced garlic to the pot and cook for an additional minute until fragrant.

3. Add diced potatoes to the pot and cook for 3-4 minutes, allowing them to slightly brown.

4. Pour in the vegetable or chicken broth, dried thyme, and red pepper flakes if using. Bring the soup to a boil, then reduce the heat to low and let it simmer, covered, for about 15-20 minutes or until the potatoes are tender.

5. Add chopped kale to the pot and simmer for an additional 5-7 minutes until the kale is wilted.

6. Season the soup with salt and pepper to taste. Adjust the seasoning as needed.

7. Before serving, ladle the Fresh Kale Garlic Soup into bowls.

8. Optionally, sprinkle each serving with grated Parmesan cheese.

9. Serve with crusty bread if desired.

Sweetcorn Soup

Ingredients:

- 2 cups sweetcorn kernels (fresh or frozen)
- 1 onion, finely chopped
- 2 cloves garlic, minced
- 1 carrot, peeled and diced
- 4 cups vegetable or chicken broth
- 1 potato, peeled and diced
- 1 cup milk
- 2 tablespoons butter
- 2 tablespoons all-purpose flour
- 1/2 teaspoon dried thyme
- Salt and pepper to taste
- Fresh chives or parsley, chopped (for garnish)

Instructions:

1. In a large pot, melt butter over medium heat. Add chopped onion and cook until softened, about 3-4 minutes.

2. Add minced garlic to the pot and cook for an additional minute until fragrant.

3. Sprinkle the flour over the onion and garlic mixture, stirring constantly to create a roux. Cook for 2-3 minutes to eliminate the raw flour taste.

4. Slowly pour in the vegetable or chicken broth, stirring continuously to avoid lumps. Bring the mixture to a gentle boil.

5. Add diced potatoes and carrots to the pot. Simmer for about 10-15 minutes or until the vegetables are tender.

6. Stir in sweetcorn kernels and dried thyme. Cook for an additional 5-7 minutes.

7. Using an immersion blender, blend the soup until it reaches your desired consistency. If you don't have an immersion blender, transfer a portion of the soup to a blender and blend until smooth, then return it to the pot.

8. Stir in milk and season the soup with salt and pepper to taste. Adjust the seasoning as needed.

9. Let the Sweetcorn Soup simmer for another 5 minutes to heat through.

10. Ladle the soup into bowls and garnish with fresh chives or parsley.

Creamy Spinach Soup with Quinoa

Ingredients:
- 1 cup quinoa, rinsed
- 2 tablespoons olive oil

- 1 onion, finely chopped
- 3 cloves garlic, minced
- 6 cups vegetable broth
- 1 potato, peeled and diced
- 1 carrot, peeled and diced
- 4 cups fresh spinach, chopped
- 1 cup milk (or non-dairy milk for a vegan option)
- 2 tablespoons butter (or olive oil for a vegan option)
- 2 tablespoons all-purpose flour (or a gluten-free alternative)
- 1/2 teaspoon ground nutmeg
- Salt and pepper to taste
- Fresh lemon juice (optional, for serving)
- Grated Parmesan cheese (optional, for serving)

Instructions:

1. In a medium saucepan, combine quinoa with 2 cups of water. Bring to a boil, then reduce heat to low, cover, and simmer for 15-20 minutes or until the quinoa is cooked and water is absorbed. Set aside.

2. In a large pot, heat olive oil over medium heat. Add chopped onion and cook until softened, about 3-4 minutes.

3. Add minced garlic to the pot and cook for an additional minute until fragrant.

4. Sprinkle the flour over the onion and garlic mixture, stirring constantly to create a roux. Cook for 2-3 minutes to eliminate the raw flour taste.

5. Slowly pour in the vegetable broth, stirring continuously to avoid lumps. Bring the mixture to a gentle boil.

6. Add diced potatoes and carrots to the pot. Simmer for about 10-15 minutes or until the vegetables are tender.

7. Stir in chopped spinach and cook for an additional 3-5 minutes until the spinach is wilted.

8. In a separate small saucepan, melt butter (or heat olive oil). Add the cooked quinoa and toss to coat.

9. Stir the quinoa into the soup mixture, and then add milk and ground nutmeg. Season with salt and pepper to taste. Adjust the seasoning as needed.

10. Let the Creamy Spinach Soup with Quinoa simmer for another 5 minutes to heat through.

11. Optionally, squeeze fresh lemon juice over the soup just before serving.
12. Ladle the soup into bowls. Optionally, sprinkle each serving with grated Parmesan cheese.

Rotisserie Chicken Noodle Soup

Ingredients:

- 1 rotisserie chicken, meat shredded (about 3-4 cups)
- 1 tablespoon olive oil
- 1 onion, finely chopped
- 2 carrots, peeled and sliced
- 2 celery stalks, sliced
- 3 cloves garlic, minced
- 8 cups chicken broth
- 2 bay leaves
- 1 teaspoon dried thyme
- 1 teaspoon dried rosemary
- Salt and pepper to taste
- 2 cups egg noodles
- 1 cup frozen peas
- Fresh parsley, chopped (for garnish)
- Lemon wedges (optional, for serving)

Instructions:

1. In a large pot, heat olive oil over medium heat. Add chopped onion, carrots, and celery. Sauté until the vegetables are softened, about 5 minutes.

2. Add minced garlic to the pot and cook for an additional minute until fragrant.

3. Pour in the chicken broth, add the bay leaves, dried thyme, dried rosemary, and shredded rotisserie chicken. Bring the soup to a boil, then reduce the heat to low and let it simmer, covered, for about 15-20 minutes to allow the flavors to meld.

4. Season the soup with salt and pepper to taste. Adjust the seasoning as needed.

5. Add egg noodles to the pot and cook according to the package instructions until they are al dente.

6. Stir in frozen peas and cook for an additional 3-5 minutes until the peas are heated through.

7. Before serving, remove the bay leaves and discard them.

8. Ladle the Rotisserie Chicken Noodle Soup into bowls. Garnish with fresh chopped parsley.

9. Optionally, serve with lemon wedges on the side for a burst of citrus flavor.

Cream of Crab Soup

Ingredients:

- 1/2 cup unsalted butter
- 1/2 cup all-purpose flour
- 1 small onion, finely chopped
- 2 stalks celery, finely chopped
- 1 red bell pepper, finely chopped
- 3 cloves garlic, minced
- 4 cups chicken broth
- 2 cups half-and-half
- 1 teaspoon Old Bay seasoning
- 1/2 teaspoon dry mustard
- 1/2 teaspoon Worcestershire sauce
- 1/4 teaspoon cayenne pepper
- Salt and black pepper to taste
- 1 pound lump crab meat, picked over for shells
- 1/2 cup sherry wine (optional, for serving)
- Fresh parsley, chopped (for garnish)
- Old Bay seasoning (for garnish)

Instructions:

1. In a large pot, melt the butter over medium heat. Add the finely chopped onion, celery, and red bell pepper. Cook until the vegetables are softened, about 5-7 minutes.

2. Sprinkle the flour over the vegetables, stirring continuously to create a roux. Cook for 2-3 minutes to eliminate the raw flour taste.

3. Gradually whisk in the chicken broth to ensure a smooth consistency. Continue whisking until the mixture thickens.

4. Stir in minced garlic and cook for an additional minute until fragrant.

5. Pour in the half-and-half, Old Bay seasoning, dry mustard, Worcestershire sauce, cayenne pepper, salt, and black pepper. Stir to combine.

6. Allow the soup to simmer for about 10-15 minutes, stirring occasionally.

7. Gently fold in the lump crab meat, being careful not to break up the crab too much. Cook for an additional 5 minutes to heat through.

8. Taste the soup and adjust the seasoning as needed.

9. Ladle the Cream of Crab Soup into bowls. Optionally, drizzle each serving with sherry wine.

10. Garnish with fresh chopped parsley and a sprinkle of Old Bay seasoning.

Roasted Cauliflower & Potato Curry Soup

Ingredients:

- 1 head cauliflower, cut into florets
- 2 large potatoes, peeled and diced
- 1 onion, finely chopped
- 3 cloves garlic, minced
- 2 tablespoons curry powder
- 1 teaspoon ground cumin
- 1 teaspoon ground coriander
- 1/2 teaspoon turmeric
- 1/2 teaspoon cayenne pepper (adjust to taste)
- 4 cups vegetable broth
- 1 can (14 oz) coconut milk
- 2 tablespoons olive oil
- Salt and pepper to taste
- Fresh cilantro, chopped (for garnish)
- Lime wedges (for serving)

Instructions:

1. Preheat the oven to 400°F (200°C). Place cauliflower florets and diced potatoes on a baking sheet. Drizzle with olive oil and season with salt and pepper. Roast in the oven for about 25-30 minutes or until the vegetables are golden and tender.

2. In a large pot, heat olive oil over medium heat. Add chopped onion and cook until softened, about 3-4 minutes.

3. Add minced garlic to the pot and cook for an additional minute until fragrant.

4. Stir in curry powder, ground cumin, ground coriander, turmeric, and cayenne pepper. Cook for 1-2 minutes to toast the spices.

5. Add roasted cauliflower and potatoes to the pot. Pour in vegetable broth and bring the mixture to a boil. Reduce the heat to low and let it simmer, covered, for about 10-15 minutes.

6. Use an immersion blender to puree the soup until smooth. If you don't have an immersion blender, transfer the soup in batches to a blender and blend until smooth, then return it to the pot.

7. Stir in coconut milk and season the soup with salt and pepper to taste. Adjust the seasoning as needed.

8. Allow the Roasted Cauliflower & Potato Curry Soup to simmer for an additional 5 minutes to heat through.

9. Ladle the soup into bowls. Garnish with fresh chopped cilantro.

10. Serve with lime wedges on the side for squeezing over the soup.

Red Lentil and Tomato Soup

Ingredients:

- 1 cup red lentils, rinsed and drained
- 1 onion, finely chopped
- 2 carrots, peeled and diced
- 3 cloves garlic, minced
- 1 can (14 oz) diced tomatoes
- 6 cups vegetable broth
- 1 teaspoon ground cumin
- 1 teaspoon ground coriander
- 1/2 teaspoon smoked paprika
- 1 bay leaf
- Salt and pepper to taste

- 2 tablespoons olive oil
- Fresh cilantro, chopped (for garnish)
- Lemon wedges (for serving)

Instructions:

1. In a large pot, heat olive oil over medium heat. Add chopped onion, carrots, and garlic. Sauté until the vegetables are softened, about 5 minutes.

2. Add ground cumin, ground coriander, and smoked paprika to the pot. Cook for 1-2 minutes to toast the spices.

3. Pour in the red lentils, diced tomatoes (with their juice), and vegetable broth. Add the bay leaf. Bring the soup to a boil, then reduce the heat to low and let it simmer, covered, for about 20-25 minutes or until the lentils are tender.

4. Season the soup with salt and pepper to taste. Adjust the seasoning as needed.

5. Before serving, remove the bay leaf and discard it.

6. Use an immersion blender to partially blend the soup, leaving some lentils and vegetables for texture. If you prefer a smoother soup, blend to your desired consistency.

7. Ladle the Red Lentil and Tomato Soup into bowls. Garnish with fresh chopped cilantro.

8. Serve with lemon wedges on the side for squeezing over the soup.

Spinach Soup

Ingredients:

- 1 tablespoon olive oil
- 1 onion, finely chopped
- 2 cloves garlic, minced
- 1 potato, peeled and diced
- 6 cups vegetable broth
- 1 bay leaf
- 1 teaspoon dried thyme
- 1/2 teaspoon ground nutmeg
- Salt and pepper to taste
- 8 cups fresh spinach, chopped
- 1 cup milk (or non-dairy milk for a vegan option)
- 2 tablespoons butter (or olive oil for a vegan option)
- Fresh lemon juice (optional, for serving)
- Greek yogurt or sour cream (optional, for serving)

Instructions:

1. In a large pot, heat olive oil over medium heat. Add chopped onion and cook until softened, about 3-4 minutes.

2. Add minced garlic to the pot and cook for an additional minute until fragrant.

3. Add diced potatoes to the pot and cook for 3-4 minutes, allowing them to slightly brown.

4. Pour in the vegetable broth, add the bay leaf, dried thyme, ground nutmeg, salt, and pepper. Bring the soup to a boil, then reduce the heat to low and let it simmer, covered, for about 15-20 minutes or until the potatoes are tender.

5. Stir in chopped fresh spinach and cook for an additional 3-5 minutes until the spinach is wilted.

6. Use an immersion blender to blend the soup until smooth. If you don't have an immersion blender, transfer a portion of the soup to a blender and blend until smooth, then return it to the pot.

7. In a small saucepan, melt butter (or heat olive oil). Stir in milk and warm the mixture without boiling.

8. Stir the warm milk mixture into the soup, and adjust the seasoning as needed.

9. Optionally, squeeze fresh lemon juice into the soup just before serving.

10. Ladle the Spinach Soup into bowls. Optionally, top each serving with a dollop of Greek yogurt or sour cream.

"Nutrient-rich meals provide the foundation for my vibrant energy."

"I find joy in creating and savoring meals that support my digestive system."

CHAPTER 12: DINING OUT AND TRAVELING ON A NO GALLBLADDER DIET

Dining out and traveling while on a no gallbladder diet necessitates careful planning in order to maintain a healthy lifestyle. Individuals who do not have a gallbladder must make dietary changes because it is essential for fat digestion.

Here's a step-by-step method to navigating these situations:

1. Select Lean Proteins: Choose lean protein sources such grilled chicken, fish, or lean cuts of meat. These are more easily digestible and place less load on your digestive system.

2. Embrace Healthy Fats: Include more healthy fats in your diet, such as avocados, olive oil, and almonds, which are easier to digest without the help of the gallbladder. To avoid overburdening your digestive system, keep meal amounts in mind.

3. Limit your intake of fried and greasy foods: Fried and greasy foods can be difficult for folks who do not have a gallbladder. When dining out, choose baked, grilled, or steamed dishes over fried options to limit your intake of hard-to-digest fats.

4. Portion Control: Smaller, more frequent meals can be gentler on the digestive system than large, heavy ones. Pack healthy snacks like almonds, seeds, or fruit when traveling to help manage your eating routine.

5. Choose Fiber-Rich Foods: Consume fiber-rich foods such as fruits, vegetables, and whole grains. Fiber assists digestion and regulates bowel motions, which might be good for people who have a weakened digestive system.

6. Maintain Adequate Hydration: Adequate hydration is critical for general health and digestion. When traveling, bring a reusable water bottle and choose for water or herbal teas over sugary or caffeinated beverages.

7. Research Restaurants in Advance: Before going out to eat, investigate restaurants in the neighborhood to identify ones that provide healthier options. Look for menus that feature grilled or steamed meals, and don't be afraid to inquire about preparation methods.

8. Communicate Dietary requirements: When ordering at a restaurant, make it clear to the waitress about your dietary requirements. Most restaurants are accommodating and can adjust dishes to meet your requirements.

9. Plan Ahead: When traveling, plan your meals ahead of time. Determine acceptable eateries or prepare some meals to take with you. This proactive strategy ensures that you have access to appropriate foods, which is especially important in places with limited dining options.

TIPS FOR TRAVELING WHILE MAINTAINING DIETARY NEEDS

Traveling while adhering to dietary requirements, for those without a gallbladder, necessitates meticulous planning to guarantee a healthy and comfortable vacation.

Here's a detailed guide with ideas for traveling while considering your dietary needs:

1. Plan Ahead: Plan ahead of time by researching destination possibilities and dining venues. To make informed decisions while traveling, look for restaurants that provide healthier and no gallbladder-friendly options.

2. Pack Snacks: Bring snacks that meet your dietary requirements. To keep healthy options readily available, consider nuts, seeds, whole grain crackers, or fresh fruits.

3. Keep Hydrated: Hydration is essential, especially when traveling. Carry a reusable water bottle with you and drink enough water to aid digestion and overall well-being.

4. Choose No Gallbladder-Friendly Foods: Choose meals high in lean protein, healthy fats, and fiber. Look for grilled proteins, salads, and vegetable-based foods to help digestion without a gallbladder.

5. Limit your intake of processed foods: Reduce your consumption of processed and highly processed foods. For a more nutrient-dense and digestive-friendly diet, stick to whole, unprocessed foods.

6. Communication is Key: Inform airline personnel, hotels, and restaurants about your dietary restrictions. Many establishments are willing to accommodate special demands if they are informed ahead of time.

7. Explore Local Grocery Stores: Visit local grocery shops for fresh vegetables, lean proteins, and other goods that fit your nutritional needs. This gives you control over your eating choices.

8. Be Wary of Alcohol Consumption: If you must drink alcohol, do it in moderation. Excessive alcohol consumption can be difficult to digest, especially for people who do not have a gallbladder.

9. Consider Time Zones: Gradually adjust your eating routine to the local time zone. This aids in the adaptation of your digestive system, minimizing the likelihood of stomach discomfort.

10. Pack No Gallbladder-Friendly Snack Bags: Prepare small snack bags filled with no gallbladder-friendly foods including raw veggies, fruits, and a variety of nuts. These can be useful on long flights or road excursions.

11. Choose Customizable Meals: Choose places that provide customisable meals when dining out. This allows you to customize your order to match your exact dietary requirements.

12. Maintain Physical Activity: Incorporate physical activity into your trip plans. This can help with digestion and alleviate any discomfort caused by dietary changes.

CONCLUSION

In conclusion, the "No Gallbladder Diet Cookbook" is a guide that empowers those who have had their gallbladder removed to embrace a healthy lifestyle through a variety of low-fat recipes and digestive-friendly meals. This priceless resource not only tackles the difficulties of living without a gallbladder, but it also promotes a revitalized sense of well-being by supporting food choices that support good digestion.

This cookbook encourages a conscious approach to nutrition via skillfully picked dishes that offer delectable alternatives without sacrificing intestinal comfort. The cookbook caters to the special needs of persons who have had gallbladder removal surgery, preventing discomfort and enhancing overall digestive health by emphasizing on low-fat options.

Aside from the recipes, the cookbook provides crucial insights into the subtleties of a gallbladder-free lifestyle. From food changes to lifestyle suggestions, readers receive a comprehensive understanding of how to navigate and thrive after gallbladder removal.

In essence, the "No Gallbladder Diet Cookbook" is a companion for individuals seeking a healthy and joyful life after gallbladder surgery. This guide opens the way for a healthier, more joyful lifestyle with nutritional culinary creativity—one that celebrates nourishing the body while acknowledging and responding to its individual demands.

HAPPY COOKING!

USEFUL RESOURCES

NO GALLBLADDER DIET SHOPPING LIST

It's critical to make mindful choices when following a no-gallbladder diet to improve digestion and avoid discomfort.

Here's a thorough shopping list for people who don't have a gallbladder:

1. **Lean Proteins:**
   - Skinless poultry
   - Lean cuts of beef or pork
   - Fish (especially fatty fish like salmon for omega-3 fatty acids)

2. **Healthy Fats:**
   - Olive oil
   - Avocado oil
   - Flaxseed oil
   - Fatty fish (salmon, mackerel, sardines)

3. **Low-Fat Dairy:**
   - Skim or low-fat milk
   - Greek yogurt (low-fat)

- Cottage cheese (low-fat)

4. **Fruits:**
   - Berries (strawberries, blueberries, raspberries)
   - Apples (without the skin)
   - Bananas
   - Kiwi

5. **Vegetables:**
   - Leafy greens (spinach, kale, lettuce)
   - Zucchini
   - Cucumber
   - Carrots (cooked or shredded)

6. **Whole Grains:**
   - Quinoa
   - Brown rice
   - Oats
   - Whole wheat bread or pasta (in moderation)

7. **Herbs and Spices:**
   - Ginger
   - Turmeric
   - Cilantro
   - Mint

8. **Nuts and Seeds:**
    - Almonds (in moderation)
    - Chia seeds
    - Flaxseeds

9. **Beverages:**
    - Water (stay well-hydrated)
    - Herbal teas (peppermint, chamomile)
    - Freshly squeezed juices (in moderation)

10. **Avoid or Limit:**
    - Fried and greasy foods
    - Full-fat dairy
    - Spicy foods
    - Highly processed foods
    - Carbonated beverages

28-DAY MEAL PLAN

DAY 1

BREAKFAST: Oatmeal with sliced strawberries and a dollop of low-fat yogurt (p. 68)

LUNCH: Grilled chicken breast with quinoa and steamed broccoli (p. 74)

DINNER: Baked fish with a side of roasted sweet potatoes and mixed vegetables (p. 122)

SNACK: Greek yogurt with a handful of mixed nuts (p. 193)

DAY 2

BREAKFAST: Whole grain toast with avocado slices and a fruit salad (p. 63)

LUNCH: Turkey and vegetable stir-fry with brown rice (p. 77)

DINNER: Salmon filet with asparagus and quinoa (p. 125)

SNACK: Chia seed pudding with berries (p. 179)

DAY 3

BREAKFAST: Buckwheat pancakes with mixed berries and a side of Greek yogurt (p. 29)

LUNCH: Grilled shrimp salad with mixed greens, cherry tomatoes, and a light olive oil vinaigrette (p. 79)

DINNER: Stir-fried tofu with broccoli and quinoa (p. 127)

SNACK: Sliced apple with almond butter (p. 185)

DAY 4

BREAKFAST: Smoothie with spinach, banana, chia seeds, and a scoop of protein powder (p. 33)

LUNCH: Lentil soup with a side of whole grain roll (p. 82)

DINNER: Baked chicken thighs with sweet potato wedges and green beans (p. 130)

SNACK: Cottage cheese with pineapple chunks (p. 192)

DAY 5

BREAKFAST: Whole grain cereal with sliced peaches and low-fat milk (p. 38)

LUNCH: Turkey lettuce wraps with hummus and cucumber (p. 84)

DINNER: Grilled cod with quinoa pilaf and roasted Brussels sprouts (p. 133)

SNACK: Handful of walnuts and a small bunch of grapes (p. 198)

DAY 6

BREAKFAST: Scrambled eggs with spinach and whole grain toast (p. 42)

LUNCH: Quinoa salad with cherry tomatoes, feta cheese, and a lemon-tahini dressing (p. 87)

DINNER: Baked trout with lemon and dill, served with brown rice and steamed asparagus (p. 136)

SNACK: Carrot sticks with hummus (p. 188)

DAY 7

BREAKFAST: Overnight oats with sliced banana and a sprinkle of flaxseeds (p. 36)

LUNCH: Grilled chicken Caesar salad with cherry tomatoes and whole grain croutons (p. 89)

DINNER: Stir-fried beef with colorful bell peppers and brown rice (p. 139)

SNACK: A handful of mixed berries with a dollop of low-fat yogurt (p. 174)

DAY 8

BREAKFAST: Whole grain waffles with fresh berries and a drizzle of honey (p. 59)

LUNCH: Chickpea and vegetable curry with quinoa (p. 95)

DINNER: Baked turkey meatballs with zucchini noodles and marinara sauce (p. 141)

SNACK: Edamame with a sprinkle of sea salt (p. 175)

DAY 9

BREAKFAST: Spinach and feta omelet with whole grain toast (p. 51)

LUNCH: Shrimp and avocado salad with mixed greens and a lime-cilantro dressing (p. 98)

DINNER: Grilled lean pork chops with sweet potato mash and green beans (p. 144)

SNACK: Mixed nuts and dried fruit trail mix (p. 184)

DAY 10

BREAKFAST: Greek yogurt parfait with granola and mixed fruit (p. 67)

LUNCH: Quinoa-stuffed bell peppers with black beans and corn (p. 100)

DINNER: Baked chicken with lemon and rosemary, served with wild rice and roasted vegetables (p. 147)

SNACK: Carrot and cucumber sticks with tzatziki (p. 178)

DAY 11

BREAKFAST: Smoothie bowl with mango, kiwi, and a sprinkle of pumpkin seeds (p. 57)

LUNCH: Turkey and vegetable stir-fry with brown rice (p. 77)

DINNER: Grilled salmon with quinoa salad (tomatoes, cucumber, and fresh herbs) (p. 150)

SNACK: Sliced apple with almond butter (p. 185)

DAY 12

BREAKFAST: Whole grain bagel with smoked salmon, cream cheese, and sliced tomatoes (p. 41)

LUNCH: Turkey and vegetable kebabs with a side of hummus and whole wheat pita (p. 92)

DINNER: Baked cod with a citrus glaze, served with sweet potato wedges and steamed broccoli (p. 152)

SNACK: Cottage cheese with pineapple chunks (p. 192)

DAY 13

BREAKFAST: Scrambled tofu with sautéed spinach and whole grain toast (p. 46)

LUNCH: Quinoa-stuffed bell peppers with black beans and corn (p. 100)

DINNER: Grilled chicken breast with a side of wild rice and roasted Brussels sprouts (p. 155)

SNACK: A handful of mixed berries with a dollop of low-fat yogurt (p. 174)

DAY 14

BREAKFAST: Oat bran muffins with blueberries and a side of low-fat yogurt (p. 55)

LUNCH: Stir-fried shrimp with broccoli and snap peas, served over brown rice (p. 102)

DINNER: Baked turkey cutlets with a cranberry-orange glaze, quinoa, and roasted sweet potatoes (p. 158)

SNACK: Greek yogurt with a handful of mixed nuts (p. 193)

DAY 15

BREAKFAST: Chia seed pudding with mango chunks and a handful of pistachios (p. 72)

LUNCH: Chicken and vegetable lettuce wraps with a side of sliced cucumber (p. 104)

DINNER: Baked trout with lemon and dill, served with brown rice and steamed asparagus (p. 136)

SNACK: Sliced bell peppers with hummus (p. 170)

DAY 16

BREAKFAST: Whole grain toast with avocado slices and a fruit salad (p. 63)

LUNCH: Quinoa and kale salad with roasted chickpeas and a lemon-tahini dressing (p. 107)

DINNER: Grilled lean pork chops with sweet potato mash and green beans (p. 144)

SNACK: Mixed nuts and dried apricots (p. 197)

DAY 17

BREAKFAST: Greek yogurt smoothie with mixed berries and a tablespoon of flaxseeds (p. 48)

LUNCH: Baked chicken thighs with a side of barley and roasted vegetables (p. 110)

DINNER: Stir-fried tofu with bok choy and brown rice (p. 161)

SNACK: Sliced apple with a small portion of cheese (p. 196)

DAY 18

BREAKFAST: Spinach and feta omelet with whole grain toast (p. 51)

LUNCH: Lentil soup with a side of whole grain roll (p. 82)

DINNER: Grilled salmon with quinoa salad (tomatoes, cucumber, and fresh herbs) (p. 150)

SNACK: Carrot and cucumber sticks with tzatziki (p. 178)

DAY 19

BREAKFAST: Overnight chia seed oats with pineapple and shredded coconut (p. 49)

LUNCH: Turkey and vegetable wraps with whole wheat tortillas (p. 113)

DINNER: Baked cod with a citrus glaze, served with sweet potato wedges and steamed broccoli (p. 152)

SNACK: Cottage cheese with pineapple chunks (p. 192)

DAY 20

BREAKFAST: Buckwheat pancakes with mixed berries and a side of Greek yogurt (p. 29)

LUNCH: Chickpea and vegetable curry with quinoa (p. 95)

DINNER: Grilled chicken breast with a side of wild rice and roasted Brussels sprouts (p. 155)

SNACK: Handful of walnuts and a small bunch of grapes (p. 198)

DAY 21

BREAKFAST: Smoothie bowl with mango, kiwi, and a sprinkle of pumpkin seeds (p. 57)

LUNCH: Lentil and vegetable stir-fry with quinoa (p. 115)

DINNER: Grilled shrimp with a side of wild rice and roasted Brussels sprouts (p. 164)

SNACK: Sliced apple with almond butter (p. 185)

DAY 22

BREAKFAST: Whole grain bagel with smoked salmon, cream cheese, and sliced tomatoes (p. 41)

LUNCH: Turkey and vegetable kebabs with a side of hummus and whole wheat pita (p. 92)

DINNER: Baked cod with a citrus glaze, served with sweet potato wedges and steamed broccoli (p. 152)

SNACK: Cottage cheese with pineapple chunks (p. 192)

DAY 23

BREAKFAST: Scrambled tofu with sautéed spinach and whole grain toast (p. 46)

LUNCH: Quinoa and black bean salad with corn, cherry tomatoes, and avocado (p. 118)

DINNER: Grilled chicken breast with a side of wild rice and roasted Brussels sprouts (p. 155)

SNACK: A handful of mixed berries with a dollop of low-fat yogurt (p. 174)

DAY 24

BREAKFAST: Oat bran muffins with blueberries and a side of low-fat yogurt (p. 55)

LUNCH: Stir-fried shrimp with broccoli and snap peas, served over brown rice (p. 102)

DINNER: Baked turkey cutlets with a cranberry-orange glaze, quinoa, and roasted sweet potatoes (p. 158)

SNACK: Greek yogurt with a handful of mixed nuts (p. 193)

DAY 25

BREAKFAST: Chia seed pudding with mango chunks and a handful of pistachios (p. 72)

LUNCH: Chicken and vegetable lettuce wraps with a side of sliced cucumber (p. 104)

DINNER: Baked trout with lemon and dill, served with brown rice and steamed asparagus (p. 136)

SNACK: Sliced bell peppers with hummus (p. 170)

DAY 26

BREAKFAST: Whole grain toast with avocado slices fruit salad (p. 63)

LUNCH: Quinoa and kale salad with roasted chickpeas and a lemon-tahini dressing (p. 107)

DINNER: Grilled lean pork chops with sweet potato mash and green beans (p. 144)

SNACK: Mixed nuts and dried apricots (p. 197)

DAY 27

BREAKFAST: Greek yogurt smoothie with mixed berries and a tablespoon of flaxseeds (p. 48)

LUNCH: Baked chicken thighs with a side of barley and roasted vegetables (p. 110)

DINNER: Stir-fried tofu with bok choy and brown rice (p. 161)

SNACK: Sliced apple with a small portion of cheese (p. 196)

DAY 28

BREAKFAST: Overnight chia seed oats with pineapple and shredded coconut (p. 49)

LUNCH: Turkey and vegetable wraps with whole wheat tortillas (p. 113)

DINNER: Grilled salmon with quinoa salad (tomatoes, cucumber, and fresh herbs) (p. 150)

SNACK: Carrot and cucumber sticks with tzatziki (p. 178

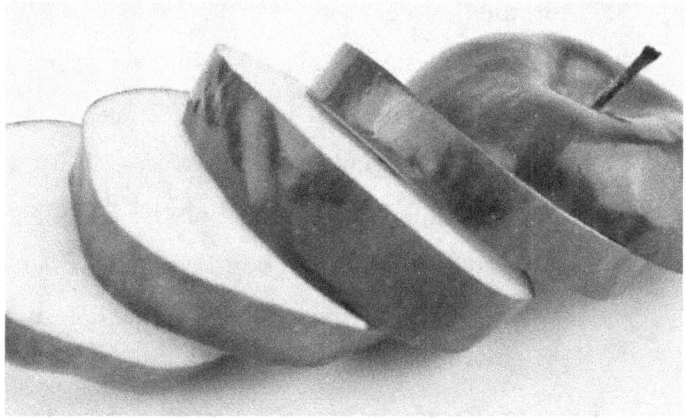

EXERCISE FOR NO GALLBLADDER HEALTH

Individuals who do not have a gallbladder can focus on exercises that improve overall health without overtaxing the digestive system.

Here's a more detailed breakdown:

1. **Aerobic Exercises:**
   - Walking: A great low-impact exercise that improves digestion and cardiovascular health.
   - Swimming: It is easy on the joints and delivers a full-body workout without putting too much strain on the digestive system.
   - Cycling: Another low-impact method for improving cardiovascular fitness.

2. **Strength Training:**
   - Focus on Core Strength: Core muscle strengthening can help to keep the spine stable and improve posture without triggering digestive problems.

- Bodyweight Exercises: Squats, lunges, and push-ups can help you maintain muscular mass and boost your metabolism.

3. **Flexibility and Stretching:**
   - Yoga: It aids in the improvement of flexibility, balance, and relaxation. Choose positions that do not place undue strain on the abdomen.
   - Pilates: Focuses on core strength and overall flexibility, often through controlled movements.

4. **Considerations:**
   - Moderation is Key: Exercises that are too intense may strain the digestive system. Aim for a well-rounded routine that includes both aerobics and strength training.
   - Listen to Your Body: If any workout produces discomfort or agony, it is critical to modify or discontinue it.

"Every recipe is a step towards a thriving, gallbladder-free life."

"I appreciate the journey of discovering and enjoying new, healthy foods."

NO GALLBLADDER DIET MEAL PLANNER

PLANNER

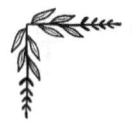

WEEKLY MEAL PLANNER

MONDAY	TUESDAY	WEDNESDAY

THURSDAY	FRIDAY	SHOPPING LIST

SATURDAY	SUNDAY

Notes:

WEEKLY MEAL PLANNER

MONDAY	TUESDAY	WEDNESDAY

THURSDAY	FRIDAY	SHOPPING LIST

SATURDAY	SUNDAY

Notes:

WEEKLY MEAL PLANNER

MONDAY	TUESDAY	WEDNESDAY

THURSDAY	FRIDAY	SHOPPING LIST

SATURDAY	SUNDAY

Notes:

WEEKLY MEAL
PLANNER

MONDAY	TUESDAY	WEDNESDAY

THURSDAY	FRIDAY	SHOPPING LIST

SATURDAY	SUNDAY

Notes:

WEEKLY MEAL PLANNER

MONDAY	TUESDAY	WEDNESDAY

THURSDAY	FRIDAY	SHOPPING LIST

SATURDAY	SUNDAY

Notes:

WEEKLY MEAL
PLANNER

MONDAY	TUESDAY	WEDNESDAY

THURSDAY	FRIDAY	SHOPPING LIST

SATURDAY	SUNDAY

Notes:

WEEKLY MEAL PLANNER

MONDAY	**TUESDAY**	**WEDNESDAY**

THURSDAY	**FRIDAY**	**SHOPPING LIST**

SATURDAY	**SUNDAY**

Notes:

WEEKLY MEAL PLANNER

MONDAY	TUESDAY	WEDNESDAY

THURSDAY	FRIDAY	SHOPPING LIST

SATURDAY	SUNDAY

Notes: